HORSES & STRESS

All photos by Kathleen Camp

Published in the United States by 14 Hands Press,

an imprint of Camp Horse Camp, LLC

www.14handspress.com

Library of Congress Control Number: 2013903890

Library of Congress subject headings

Camp, Joe

Horses & Stress / by Joe Camp

Horses

Human-animal relationships

Horses-health, Diet

Hoof Care, Training

The Soul of a Horse: Life Lessons from the Herd

ISBN 978-1-930681-15-6

First Edition

HORSES & STRESS

*Eliminating the Root Cause of
Most Health, Hoof, and
Behavior Problems*

JOE CAMP

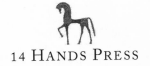

14 HANDS PRESS

Also by Joe Camp

The National Best Seller
The Soul of a Horse
Life Lessons from the Herd

The Highly Acclaimed Best Selling Sequel
Born Wild
The Soul of a Horse

Why Relationship First Works
Why and How It Changes Everything

Beginning Ground Work
Everything We've Learned About Relationship and Leadership

Training with Treats
With Relationship and Basic Training Locked In
Treats Can Be an Excellent Way to Enhance Good Communication

Why Our Horses Are Barefoot
Everything We've Learned About the
Health and Happiness of the Hoof

God Only Knows
Can You Trust Him with the Secret?

The Soul of a Horse Blogged
The Journey Continues

Horses Were Born To Be On Grass
How We Discovered the Simple But Undeniable
Truth About Grass, Sugar, Equine Diet & Lifestyle

Horses Without Grass
How We Kept Six Horses Moving and Eating Happily
Healthily on an Acre and a Half of Rocks and Dirt

Who Needs Hollywood
The Amazing Story of How Benji Became the #3 Movie of the Year

Dog On It
Everything You Need To Know About Life Is Right There At Your Feet

For Cash, Skeeter, Mariah, Mouse, Pocket,
Noelle, Malachi, Saffron, and Firestorm…
and Kathleen

All of the internet links that follow in this book are live links
in the eBook editions available at Amazon Kindle,
Barnes & Noble Nook, and Apple iBooks

"There's more to this life
than livin' and dyin'
more than just tryin'
to make it through the day."

Steven Curtis Chapman
More to this Life

CONTENTS

INTRODUCTION

I never intended to write a book, never mind several. Kathleen and I were just trying to figure out how to keep and care for a small group of horses that had somehow landed quite unexpectedly in our front yard. We were two complete neophytes who, a few short months before, didn't have a horse or a clue. So we were asking a lot of questions, and getting a lot of answers that didn't seem to make any sense. After stumbling through mistake after mistake, digging through an enormous amount of research, and spending a great deal of time with our little herd we discovered that either we were stark raving nuts or there was something very wrong in this world of horses. That's where *The Soul of a Horse* began. Thankfully for us it turned out that we weren't nuts. At least not in the clinical sense. And it was too late to turn back.

- Joe Camp

1

TRUTH

We humans are being told everyday: Curb stress and energize health and happiness.

With all the recent studies and research on the effect of emotional stress on physical issues, illness, and attitude we should all be listening.

But it's not just a message to us. It's also a message to our horses. Or rather to us *about* our horses.

How so? Horses don't have problems at the office. Or bills to pay. They don't spend hours in traffic. Or worry about losing big clients. Where's the stress?

What if God decided that we – you and I – and all the other humans on the planet – were going to live out the rest of our lives in the water. What do you think might happen?

Excuse me?

I don't mean "on" the water, like in a boat. I mean *in* the water. Up to our necks. Twenty-four hours a day. Or maybe we could get out for an hour here or an hour there, just to pay bills and do a little grocery shopping.

Would that work for us?

I wouldn't do it.

Just say for a moment that's the way things were going to be. You had no choice. Done. Splash! You would hate it, right? First and foremost because humans are not genetically designed to live in the water. So the stress associated with attempting to live like a turtle, or a salamander, or certain frogs, or even a mammal like a dolphin would, over time, be horrific. Not to mention what it might do to our bodies, muscles, skin, diet, sleep patterns, and who knows what else.

Especially over time.

Think years, decades, eons,... if we lasted that long.

I know it sounds silly but pause for a moment and *really* think about it.

Now think about your horses.

When a horse is forced to live in a manner that directly opposes the way he was genetically designed to live, the stress alone can wreak all sorts of havoc with his physical and emotional being.

So how is he genetically designed to live?

Every horse on the planet is designed to live like a wild horse.

Excuse me??

That was exactly my first reaction. But it's true. Science tells us that domestic horses and wild horses are genetically precisely the same. The horses in our back yard are really wild horses in captivity. Just like a baby tiger would be, even though his mom, grand mom, and triple-great grand mom were all born in captivity. That baby's genetics are still the same as those beasts roaming the African jungles. The scientific fact, we discovered, is that it takes between 5000 and 10,000 years to even begin to change the base genetics of any species.

Which means the horses in our back yard have been programmed for millions and millions of years to live in wide open spaces where they can see predators coming, eat small bits of grass forage around the clock up to 18 to 20 hours a day, move 8-20 miles a day, on bare feet that can flex with each step to circulate blood within the hoof capsules, live with multiple horses for safety and security, and even balance their own diets if provided with enough choices to do so.

Who knew?

Obviously not me and Kathleen when we acquired our first horses, nor the experienced experts who were advising us with phrases like: *This is the way it's always been done!* Our guys and girls all lived in a manner diametrically opposed to what their genetics were calling for. They lived in tiny little stalls where they could move at best 800 steps in a 24-hour day as opposed to the 8-20 miles a day their genetics called for. And we ultimately discovered that such a huge differential was not just affecting physical structure, it was affecting their digestion, their breathing, the health of their feet, and thereby immensely affecting their stress levels which, as medical science has finally come to realize, substantially affects all aspects of their health. Their diet was mostly sugar in a bag, which we discovered is the absolute worst thing one can feed a horse, especially a confined one. Molasses is part of virtually every packaged feed in existence. Every grain in the same bag turns to sugar the instant it gets inside the horse. And, as mentioned above, horses are genetically programmed to eat grass forage (real grass or grass hay), little bits at a time, up to 18-20 hours a day. The horse's stomach is programmed to release digestive acid around the clock. Acid that ferments grass (not sugar, not pellets, not carrots, not grain, just grass or grass hay). When that grass forage is not dribbling into the hind gut on a regular basis the acid has nothing to work on but the insides of the horse itself! Unlike humans whose digestive acid turns on and off depending upon the presence of food, the horse's digestive acid never stops. So the grass forage needs to be there. Free-choice. Around the clock.

And then there's the herd. We discovered that a horse in a stall who cannot commune with other horses gains yet another level of stress to endure. The purpose of the herd for a prey animal is safety and security. Being with other like animals is quite literally a safety net. There are more eyes to see trouble coming. And usually the dominant member of the group is also the number one watchdog. Being deprived of that comfort, at some level, breeds huge amounts of stress.

Remove all of that stress, whether human or equine, and you remove the cause of most medical and emotional issues.

For horses, just the stress of being cooped up in a stall can cause or lead to ulcers, colic, laminitis, reduced blood circulation, digestive issues and, of course, each and every stall vice in existence.

Add packaged feed filled with grain and/or sugar served up two or three times a day instead of grass or grass hay around the clock and you increase the incidence of all of the above and all sorts of other issues like insulin resistance.

Toss in the lack of movement the horse is designed to have and add metal shoes nailed to his feet that eliminate the ability for the hoof to flex which circulates the blood in the hoof capsules and up and down the legs, and all the bad stuff quickly compounds.

On and on it goes. Building the horse's immune system is the singular very best thing that can be done for a horse's health and happiness.

And building the immune system begins with eliminating stress.

Which means getting the diet, movement, feet, and blood circulation as close as your specific circumstances allow to the lifestyle the horse would be living were he or she in the wilds of the American west where he or she evolved.

I know, I know. So many have told me "I have no choice but to board my horses." Or "I simply don't have any room for them to be out." And all I can say is do the very best for your horse that your circumstances allow.

When we were in California (before the move to Tennessee) and discovered how our horses should be living this is where we started:

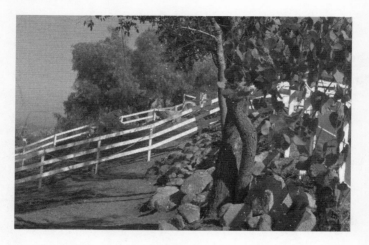

Two makeshift Paddock Paradises each barely bigger than the footprint of a barn. Each housing three horses. Not a lot of room, but at least they were out of the stalls. And they were eating grass hay around the clock spread in small piles all around the perimeter fencing and criss-crossing through the middle to stimulate movement. The dominant horse would never let #2 eat very long on a pile. So #2 would move out #3 who would go on to pile #4... and so it would go pretty much all day and night, moving around and around the paddock, except for nap times.

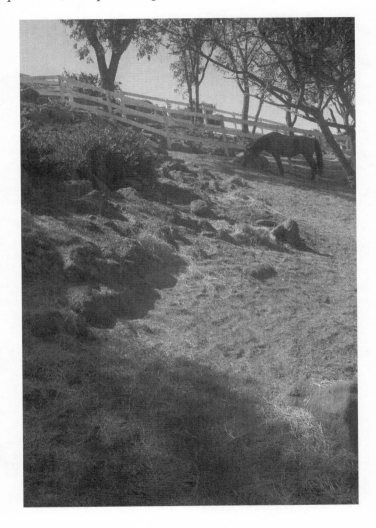

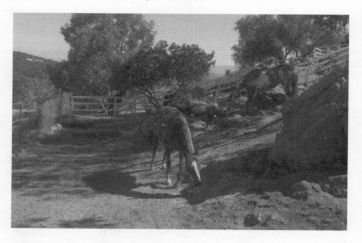

Frankly we were extremely nervous about letting the herd out into these two paddocks, scared to death that the steep hills and the rocks and boulders might cause injury... without a clue at the time that this is exactly the type of terrain that horses evolved on for millions of years out in the Great basin and Great Plains of the western USA. It didn't take long however to see that they were thriving. Happier and Healthier. We fed morning and evening. A few supplements top dressed on Triple Crown Safe Starch, a packaged forage of orchard and timothy grasses guaranteed to be less than 10% NSC (non-structured carbs which turn to sugar immediately upon entering the body), and we assured free choice grass hay around the clock by putting out morning and night, a bit more when we found it all gone, and a little less when we found some left over. Their half-covered stalls were at the top of the hill just above the above photo. Whenever a storm would blow in from the Pacific we'd move them to the stalls until the hillside dried enough to eliminate any danger of slipping.

They were doing so well that we soon began to eye the *very* steep hill behind our house. So steep it was basically worthless except as a buffer against another house getting too close. It could not be built on and basically was serving no purpose. The entire piece was a bit over two acres, but about half an acre of that was so dangerous looking we reduced our working area to approximately an acre and a half and installed an electric fence outside perimeter and another one as an inside circle that created, again, sort of a makeshift paddock paradise, only bigger than what we had originally created. In the photo below the yellow (outer) dots are the outside circle and the blue (inner) dots are the inside circle into which the horses were never allowed. A no-fly zone :).

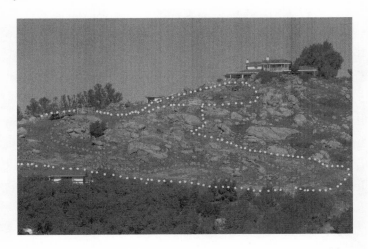

Our guess is that the final total space the herd of six
had access to was barely over an acre, but we monitored
them over one 24 hour period and estimated that they
were moving 10-12 miles a day, round and around, up
and down that hill. Eating from more than 100 little
piles of hay that we distributed all the way around,
twice a day, with our Gator. Before leaving California
we documented the entire process on video as well as
the way the horses were living and moving every day of
their lives. Watch the video on The Soul of a Horse
Channel on You Tube: **The Soul of a Horse Paddock Paradise - What We Did, How We Did It, and Why.**

The very first time we took a horse over to see how
he did, we were worried. Was it too steep? Would the
horses like it? Were there too many rocks and boulders?
Would they hurt themselves? Would they all get along
in the same pasture?

Scribbles was first.

He's the quiet one. A gorgeous paint, but charisma
is not his long suit. He's the one who was most likely to
be found standing in a corner, motionless, seemingly,
for hours. Lazy would be a merciful understatement.
He has the best *whoa* in the herd, because it's his favorite speed. No reins needed. Just sit back a little, then
hold on for the screech of tires. *Can we stop now?* is his
favorite question. He leads like it's an imposition to ask
him to move. *Oh all right, if you insist, but you have no
idea how much effort this is.*

Which is why his first venture into the natural pasture left me with my mouth hanging open in astonishment. As the halter fell away, he spun and was gone like a bullet. Racing, kicking the air, tossing his head, having the best time I'd ever seen him have. This was not a horse I had met before. He went on for a good ten minutes, with me just standing there, grinning like an idiot. I could imagine that somewhere inside those two brains he was screeching *Whoopee! I'm free! I'm free!* Finally, he trotted back over and in his own begrudging little way said thank-you. That was the beginning of a new way of life for Scribbles and his five herd mates.

A life free of stress from being confined. From eating stuff that's bad for them. A life of movement, and circulation, and good digestion. In short, a life as close as we could get to how they'd be living were they in the wild.

On barely more than an acre.

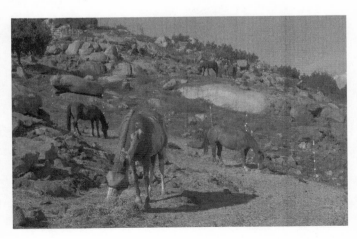

There are always ways to make their lives better. Not everyone can do what we've done. But virtually everyone can do **some**thing. There's a page on our website entitled **Happier Healthier Horses** containing short stories from folks around the world who have read one or more of our books, thought they could never achieve this better life for horses, but when they put their minds and hearts into it they discovered a way. I encourage you to read these brief tales from others who seriously love their horses. One of my favorites is from Aisha in the United Arab Republic. Please don't leave the page before reading her story. It's amazing! Here's the link:

http://thesoulofahorse.com/blog/powerful-stories-from-happier-healthier-horses/

Before we did any of this, here's it was for our horses:

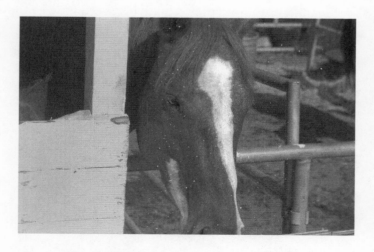

Sad eyes. Locked up. No movement. Lots of stress.

It's not that way anymore. It wasn't in California. And it's not here in middle Tennessee.

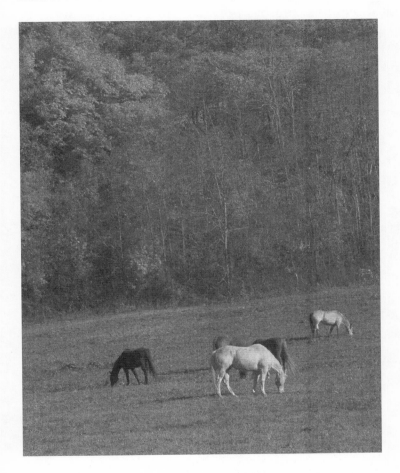

At this writing, our herd of eight is in its sixth year of being out 24/7, barefoot with the wild horse trim, eating zero sugar except what they get from the grasses of which there are multiple species from which they can choose for balance. They are getting lots of daily movement, and can use the barn breezeway as a run-in if they so choose, which they rarely do, and almost never alone. There has been no lameness, or founder, or navicular issues. No colic, no ulcers, no bad habits, no strangles, no insulin resistance.

They are eight happy and healthy horses and we are the trusted leader of each and every one of them. We almost never use a halter and lead rope except when riding, and we almost never venture out to "catch" one because a call by name will usually bring them running.

But Kathleen and I strongly encourage you to not take our word for it. Do the research. Figure it out for yourself. And see the difference that stress-free horses will add to your life. You won't be sorry you did.

2

MYTHS

But if I turn my horse loose in a pasture with other horses I'll never see him again. I'll never be able to catch him.

Myth number one.

We've heard it so many times.

There was a time when we believed it as well.

But it's simply not true *if* you begin at the beginning with your horse. If you start by putting the relationship first.

The bond first.

By giving the horse the opportunity to choose *you*. Not vice versa. That simple act makes all the difference. Allowing the horse to say *I trust you to be in my herd and be my leader.* Rather than forcing your leadership upon him.

We have eight horses. Three mustangs straight out of the wild, a rescued American Saddlebred, two Arabians, a paint and a quarter horse. Every one comes when called (most of the time :). Every one will walk with me wherever I would like to go without halter or lead rope. Every one began their journey with us by making the choice to trust us, to accept us as their leader, completely on their own. Most via Monty Roberts' Join-Up method. A couple using our No-Agenda Time. One via

Dr. Robert Miller's Foal Imprinting method. Information on all of these is available on our website or in the Resources section at the end of this book. But the difference that was made in every case by allowing the horse to choose us cannot be overstated. It's huge!

Likewise the stress to the horse created at some level by *not* allowing him that choice, by forcing your will upon him, cannot be overstated.

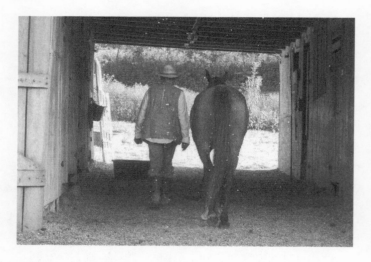

There's simply no better feeling in the world than strolling along with your horse at your side... with no strings attached. Of course, there's also the practical side. I can leave the halter and lead rope hanging on a hook when it's time to sort them for feeding. They all understand the word, "C'mon."

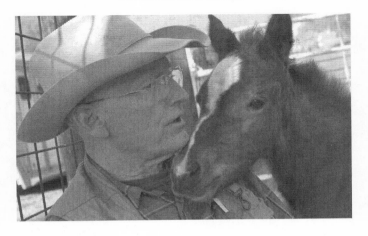

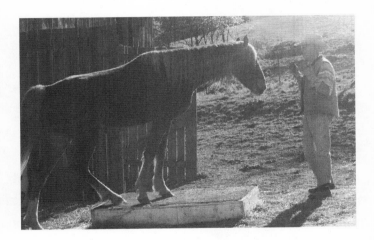

Also see the video *Relationship First* on The Soul of a Horse Channel on You Tube. For me, this video says it all. Made me cry.

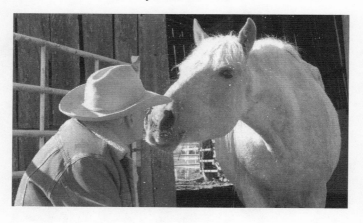

Next myth.

My horse is a jumper so he needs shoes. Or is gaited. Or is a barrel racer. Or... or... or...

German philosopher Arthur Schopenhauer said, "All truth passes through three phases. First, it is ridiculed. Second, it is violently opposed. Third, it is accepted as self-evident."

I was standing by a small arena at a local horse club event. The woman next to me was the mother of a teenager trying out a beautiful gaited pinto horse in the pen. The horse was prancing, lifting his legs high, and looking very spiffy. At one point the owner said proudly, "And he's totally barefoot."

"Wow," said the mom. "Just think what he'd look like with shoes on!"

The owner had the grace to ignore the comment. I didn't.

"Why ever would you put shoes on him? He's happy, healthy, and looks great."

"Oh, if you compete on him, he *has* to have shoes."

"Why?"

"He just has to."

"Why?"

"Well, it's probably in the rules."

"Barefoot horses compete," I said. "And win."

"Well, trust me, he needs shoes. There are special shoes that make gaited horses prance higher."

"Oh, so that's something *you* want, not something the horse wants."

There I go again, I thought. Like a reformed smoker. My presentation definitely needed work.

"Doesn't hurt him," the woman said.

I took a deep breath, swallowed the words that were threatening to escape, and handed her a card with our website on it, suggesting that she look at some of the new research documented there on how shoes affect the health of a horse's hoof. Then, I mustered a friendly smile and left.

I told Kathleen the story.

"We're going to lose every friend we have if you don't shut up," she said.

"I never saw this woman before," I whimpered. "She's not a friend."

"You know what I mean. People don't want to hear this stuff."

"Do you disagree? Is it incorrect information?"

"Of course not," she said. "But..."

"But what?"

She just looked at me for a long moment.

"Think about Skeeter," I said. "And how much happier and healthier he is since you brought him here."

"I know," she said. "I know. You're right, but it's so frustrating to have people's claws come out like they do. When you slap people in the face with the notion that they're doing something wrong, the natural reaction is always going to be to defend themselves. You do it yourself."

"I do?"

Her mouth dropped.

"*All* the time."

"When?"

"Last night when I told you that paragraph in the book was not good. You bitched, and screamed, and got ugly... and then got up this morning and changed it."

I thought about Schopenhauer's quote.

"Phase Three," I said.

We both smiled.

Katie Pontone is only eighteen years old but what follows, in her own words, is from the heart and mind of a young lady much wiser than we might expect from one with so few years under her belt:

"I have been using a certified natural trimmer on my pony jumper in New Jersey because we read your book *The Soul of a Horse* and never looked back. My pony is now the 2012 National Pony Jumper Champion because she managed the only round without fault of the top pony jumpers in the country at the national finals and **was the only barefoot one of all the pony jumpers** so I must thank you for opening my eyes to the ignorance and nonsense that trainers preach about the incredible powers of shoes.

"My pony is Wicked, who is blind in one eye, and her trimmer is Cindy Ross. Thanks to Cindy I can always count on Wicked's perfect hooves to turn tighter, gallop faster, and jump cleaner than my shod competitors. She is not only ranked number one in the United States, USEF National Pony Jumper Championships, but is the 2012 USEF *National Horse of the Year* and the USEF *Zone 2 Horse of the Year* for the Pony Jumpers. She is the number one pony jumper in the North American League and with our recent victory at the Pennsylvania National Horse Show for the 2012 North American League National Finals Wicked earned the title of the *2012 National Pony Jumper Champion*. Wicked has won at every local show she has ever been to and took home a blue first place ribbon at the 2012 Devon National Horse Show against the top pony jumpers in the country. This success was made possible through natural trimming, twenty-four hour turn out,

limited sugar intake, and ignoring everything my trainers have told me when it comes to proper horse care.

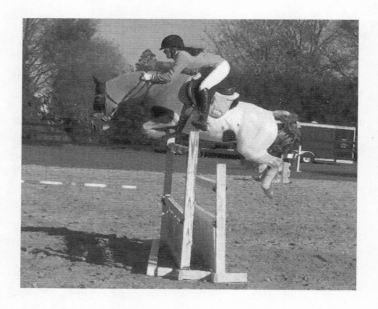

"Wicked was a terrible stopper when I first got her, she
would refuse every jump over 3'. But as her hooves
transitioned to barefoot with the wild horse model, and
she got more exercise, a healthier diet, and 24/7 turnout
the refusing came to a halt and she became the 2012
national pony jumper champion.

"I, unlike many others, win to prove a point, not to
move on to the finals or get another blue ribbon. Wicked being barefoot peaked a lot of competitors' interest.
This pony can do anything, make anyone smile, and
teach anyone to love because she absolutely loves life,
competing, and just having fun with her very own rider

since she did not have a rider that loved her for 13 years. She is the best thing to ever happen to me and she will always be my all time favorite horse." – Katie Pontone.

Read more about Katie and a host of other barefoot champions on the *Photos of Barefoot Champions* page on our website and the *Happier Healthier Horses* page.

Or just know that there isn't an event in which your horse cannot perform better barefoot with the wild horse trim.

Oh no. We've bred the hoof right off the horse. Domestic horses and wild horses are not even the same species anymore.

Another myth.

As pointed out in the previous chapter, the scientific fact is that it would take a minimum of 5000 years to even begin to change the base genetics of any species. Probably closer to 10,000 years. Scientists performed DNA sequencing on horse remains discovered in the Alaskan permafrost ranging in age from 12,000 to 28,000 years old and found that there was less than 1.2% difference when compared to the modern domestic horse in your backyard.

Millions of years of genetics could never be wiped out by a few generations of selective breeding. The reason many of these folks truly believe what they're saying is because their horse has had some sort of disorder, like lameness, for so long that they are certain he must be genetically unfit; when the problem most often lies in his metal shoes, and his tiny stall, and his diet.

Causing stress.

The most frequent argument we've heard is *My horse isn't a wild mustang, it's a domesticated horse.* As if the declaration, "He isn't running free" would somehow change the millions of years of genetics that have made him what he is. As if such a statement would make the ammonia from poop and pee eating away at his feet disappear; or cause his physical structure, which was built to be on the move constantly, to be suddenly fine with standing still twelve to twenty-four hours a day. As if it would make his respiratory system, which is built to be outside breathing fresh, clean air, suddenly find good health in breathing ammonia and high quantities of carbon dioxide in a closed environment with little circulation of fresh air. The average horse breathes 62 litres of air a minute, producing 150 litres of CO_2 per hour. And ammonia is so destructive to protein, it is actually being taken off the market in some countries.

Saying *"This isn't a wild mustang"* does not compensate for the reduced blood circulation he's suffering while wearing metal shoes standing still in a stall, Reduced circulation that, in turn, weakens the hoof by reducing the quality and quantity of horn produced by the hoof. And reduced circulation that doesn't efficiently pump blood back up the legs to the rest of the body, adding stress to the heart and affecting the immune system.

And whether mustang or domestic, it isn't healthy to eat from a bucket, feeder, or hay net hanging at table height when his body is built to eat from hoof level. Nor does being domestic negate the claustrophobia and stress he lives with at some level, caused by feeling trapped, unable to flee, alone, and bored. Never mind how willing he might be to go into the stall either because he has always been forced to, or because he knows that is where the food is.

Documented case after case confirms that these unhealthy, unhappy domestic horses can become healthy and happy again if the source of their ill health is removed, if they're given the opportunity to live as nature intended.

And they can grow a foot every bit as rock solid as those mustangs running around out there in the wild.

Next myth:
Yes, I can see that barefoot might work for some horses, but not mine. Mine's different and he needs shoes.

The Houston Mounted Police Patrol has an average of 40 horses of every breed and every background. Many of them rescued from abusive conditions.

All of them are barefoot.

All working 8-10 hours a day on the concrete, asphalt, and marble of downtown Houston.

Since the Patrol took all of their horses barefoot a few years back they have cut their vet bills in half. And reduced their accident rate from slipping to virtually nil. Read their story on our website under the menu BARE FEET.

Oh, my horse loves his stall.
Another myth.

At some level that horse is stressed. His genetics leave no choice but for this to be so.

There was a full-page ad in an issue of *Horse & Rider* magazine a couple of years ago with a big photo of a horse in a dark stall. Below the photo was this headline: *I AM CONFINED... THEREFORE I AM AT RISK.*

The subhead read: *Confinement-related stress can cause stomach ulcers in your horse – in just 5 days.*

There wasn't a word about eliminating the source of the stress or any discussion about other health problems that could be caused from a stress so tormenting that it produces stomach ulcers in five days. There was none of that because it was an ad promoting a medication for the ulcers.

An interview with Dr. Katherine Houpt, a leading animal behaviorist at Cornell University, appeared in the same issue of *Horse & Rider*. Haupt stated that this same stress is also responsible for virtually all of the so-called *stall vices*. Pawing, weaving, head bobbing, stall kicking, cribbing, wind sucking, wood chewing, and tongue lolling are all a direct result of the horse not being out with the herd, moving around, munching most of the time, with lots of roughage in his diet. Getting the horse out of the stall is all it takes. According to Dr. Houpt, these "vices" have never been observed in horses who live as mother nature intended. Considering the number of products being advertised to "solve" these problems, one has to offer kudos to *Horse & Rider* for having the courage to even publish such an article.

Humans trim their horse's coats in winter to keep them *looking good* for the show ring. This undermines the horse's ability to protect himself from the cold. Wearing blankets does the same thing. As does living in an enclosed barn, especially a climate-controlled barn. Yet this is the lifestyle of the majority of horses in the United States. Stall living also removes the horse's ability to fulfill his need to move, which affects his feet, circulation, immune system, and general health, as mentioned earlier. And it takes him away from the herd, which causes more stress. And makes him unhappy. And, as you've also read before, often leaves him standing in his own urine and poop, which also adversely affects his feet, circulation, immune system, and general health.

And so it goes.

We humans have the most extraordinary ability in the world to rationalize.

Our horses have been out 24/7 for so long that sometimes I tend to forget how other horses live. I recently visited a traditional boarding stable, a fancy one, heavily laced with dressage and show horses. I was struck with a pang of sorrow. I wanted to race through the place and pop every latch on every stall door. And pull every shoe. And rub every horse. And Join-Up with them. And listen to them.

"How often does this horse see her owner?" I asked. It was a beautiful thoroughbred cross, with very sad eyes, sort of glazed over. She was pacing, back and forth, back and forth. I stood at the stall door for a moment, but the horse never looked at me. Just paced.

"Oh, at least once every weekend. Sometimes twice."

"Who feeds her?"

"We do. Our staff."

"Who cleans the stalls?"

"Our staff. Twice a day."

"Does she get turned out?"

"Oh, absolutely. Four hours every day. Guaranteed."

"Guaranteed, huh?"

"Absolutely."

"Turned out with other horses?"

"Oh, no. She might get hurt."

"Does she have a trainer?"

"Uh huh. Comes on Tuesdays and Thursdays."

"How does the horse know who her leader is?"

"Oh, the trainer's the leader, if you want to call it that."

"And the owner?"

She looked at me like I was an idiot. I should know the answer.

"The owner is the rider in the shows," she said. "And, of course, she writes the checks."

"I see," I said, and walked on down the row of stalls.

In one way or another they were all the same. Horses penned up, away from any semblance of a herd. Showing stress in one way or another. Pacing, weaving, chewing, cribbing. One was kicking the wall. The stalls were all filled with a bedding I didn't recognize, presumably to absorb the pee, but the odor was still present, digging into their lungs. And most of them wore metal shoes.

"I notice that this one is barefoot," I said. "He doesn't have shoes."

"Strange owner," she said. "He doesn't understand that a horse has to have shoes. That's the way it is."

"Do you own horses?" I asked.

"Don't need to. Just look around."

It all reminded me of my sailing days, back when Benji was at his peak. I had a sailboat in a Fort Lauderdale marina, and I was always amazed that so many people had huge boats – mine wasn't – yet those huge boats never left the slip. The owner would pay the boarding fee, pay people to keep the boats clean, to run and service the engines, and would come down once a month and use this big, expensive yacht as a hotel room. Never go out. Never enjoy the boat, as a boat. It was just a place to hang out and sleep. And be proud of.

As frustrating as that seemed to me at the time, I suppose the good news was that it was a *boat*. An inanimate piece of fiberglass and machinery. And if the owner wanted to pour his money into that... well, it's his money.

But a horse is not a boat.

It lives and breathes, and has feelings, and worries, and a genetic system that has evolved over millions and millions of years. A boat doesn't pace and stress when it's tied in a slip. It doesn't have a herd that it should be with. It doesn't worry about being attacked by everything that blinks. A boat doesn't need to be out where it can move around all day and night. A boat doesn't feel happy or unhappy, or healthy or unhealthy because it is or isn't being ignored by its owner.

A horse does.

Our Mariah did, before she came to us.

But she doesn't feel that way anymore.

Ask her and she'll tell you which way is better.

An old cowboy on a Texas trail ride told Kathleen that all her horse wanted to do was get back to the herd. Kathleen pulled off the trail and spent some time showing this gelding that she *was* the herd. That she was a good leader. And that the horse was already there. In a herd of two. You don't really need to be a horse to be part of the herd. You just need to spend the time and effort to think like one.

And you need to care.

3

PIECING IT ALL TOGETHER

During our relatively short journey with horses we began to understand early on that, like clinician Ray Hunt always said, "What's in it for the horse?" should be the only question. And not just related to training, but to Lifestyle, Diet, and Feet. Only by understanding all of these from the horse's perspective could we begin to approach that illusory state of mind referred to as Horsemanship. We were discovering that our way to horsemanship would never be about how well we ride, or how many trophies we win, or how fast our horse runs, or how high he or she jumps.

There are many who teach relationship, riding, and training with principles of natural horsemanship. Others support the benefits of going barefoot with the wild horse trim. Still others write that your horse should eat from the ground, and live without clothes and coverings. Some promote day and night turnout, where your horses can be on the move continuously. But few have explored how dramatically one without the other can affect the horse and his well being. Few have put it all together into a single philosophy, a unified voice, a complete lifestyle change for the domesticated horse. When I gave my Cash the choice of choice and he chose me, he left me with no alternative. No longer could it be what I wanted, but rather what he needed. What fifty-two million years of genetics demanded for his long, healthy, and happy life.

But there was one problem. I had no idea what that was.

4

FEET FIRST

Shortly after our first three horses had shown up in our front yard I stumbled into wild horse research trying to uncover why Cash had come to us with shoes on his front feet but none on his back feet. We had been told that concrete and asphalt would crack and shatter any horse's hoof that was not wearing a shoe. If that were true, I needed to get shoes on his back feet right now because we had concrete and asphalt everywhere.

And I suppose I had wondered – apparently too often too loud – how wild horses had managed to exist all this time without help from humans? Could it be the wild ones might be able to teach us a thing or two?

To a prey animal like a wild horse there is nothing more important than good rock-solid feet. They travel up to thirty miles a day in search of food and water. And they run a lot from predators.

But as mentioned earlier I was being told that domesticated horses no longer had the same feet as their wild counterparts.

A domesticated hoof was destined to be weak and underdeveloped. Often sick and unhealthy. A domesticated hoof needed a metal shoe.

The American Farriers Journal reported that 95% of all domesticated horses have some sort of lameness issue. That's why they have to wear shoes, I was told.

But my Cash came to us with only *two* shoes. On the front feet. Nothing on the rear feet.

So was he half wild and half domestic?

It was worrisome that his back end would be the wild part. The kicking end.

All of this was gnawing at the edges of logic.

There is no hoof lameness in the wild. And it runs rampant throughout the domestic scene.

But unlike everyone else we had encountered, we discovered the writings of Jaime Jackson who believed that wild hoof mechanics were exactly the same as domesticated hoof mechanics, both depending upon the hoof to flex with every step taken. Like a toilet plunger. This flexing sucks an enormous amount of blood into the hoof capsule every time the hoof hits the ground; and pushes it back up the leg when the hoof leaves the ground. Like a mini-heart, pumping with every step. Among other things this keeps the hoof healthy and growing properly.

What happens when a metal shoe is nailed to the hoof?

Nothing.

No flexing.

No blood.

No function.

The curtains were parting. A veil lifting. It wasn't about whether a horse was *domesticated* or *wild*. It was about blood circulation. And the effect of that circulation – or lack of it – on the health of the hoof.

No, no, no. We've unfortunately bred the foot right off the horse.

I smiled politely. I had just read in a scientific journal that it would take a minimum of 5000 years to change the base genetics of any species. Probably more, depending upon the circumstances. A few hundred years of selective breeding could have no affect whatsoever on base genetics.

Which is why a newborn foal will still be on his feet less than an hour after being born – thinking, learning, eating – and in less than four hours be ready and able to move out with the herd to stay away from predators. Even if he's born in a stall.

The genetics haven't changed.

It's also why the stresses, illnesses, and vices caused by being confined to a stall can be solved by allowing horses to be out with each other 24/7. And it's why barefoot "domestic" horses living out with a herd, getting a lot of movement, and eating a proper diet from the ground are able to develop rock-solid hooves that have no use for metal shoes.

I called our vet.

"The shoes are coming off ," I said.

"Uhh... whose?"

"All of 'em."

Silence.

Then, "Why not try one at a time and see how it goes?"

"Nope. All six."

In a week it was done.

And not one of our horses ever looked back. I had never seen a horse smile until the day Cash's shoes were removed.

Scribbles, our paint, had hooves that were so sick that he had to grow a whole new foot, from hairline to the ground. It took eight months. But then he too was a happy camper.

How could this be? Domesticated horses need shoes because their feet are sick, soft, and unhealthy. Over and over again we were told. Or could it be that their feet are sick, soft, and unhealthy because of the metal shoes nailed to their feet restricting the circulation and eliminating the natural hydraulic-like shock absorption the intake of blood provides to protect the joints, ligaments, and tendons of the leg? I guess that's why the the country's largest mounted police patrol in Houston, Texas, have not one shoe on their forty or so horses who work all day every day on the concrete, asphalt, and marble of downtown Houston. Forty or so horses of every variety and every type of background. And not one shoe. Which eliminates the oft heard argument that some horses can go barefoot, but some cannot. All of theirs are barefoot and healthier for it. Unfortunately I didn't know any of this at the time.

If all this hadn't worked so well we would've never heard of the horse.

God and Mother Nature knew what they were doing. Horses were designed over time through trial and error to live and eat and move in certain ways; and the study of all of this could provide more incredibly valuable information about how we should be feeding, keeping, and caring for the horses we choose to associate with than has ever been understood before.

When a shoe comes off a horse that has been shod for years and years, the hoof and hoof wall are usually no longer strong and healthy. The hoof has been made unhealthy by lack of circulation because it has not been able to flex and thus circulate the blood properly throughout the hoof mechanism. And the continuing process of hammering nails into the hoof wall makes it weaker, and provides places (the nail holes) for chips and cracks to occur. Also, some hooves, if they're really in bad health, will be tender for a while after going barefoot. And the unknowing owner concludes that the tenderness means the horse needs shoes.

Not so.

The hoof will completely heal and remodel itself and grow strong new horn and hard calloused sole. This is a logical and normal process (see the Resources section at the back of the book, especially Pete Ramey's and Jaime Jackson's books and videos). It takes approximately eight months to a year for a horse to grow a new hoof, from his hairline to the ground. If properly trimmed to mimic the way wild horses' hooves trim themselves during daily wear, a worst-case scenario for a horse to acquire a completely new, rock solid, healthy foot, then, is approximately a year. Many horses are much quicker. As you read earlier, Cash was good to go from the first day his shoes came off. And a happy horse indeed. Four of our six never had a tender moment after going barefoot. One took four months to remodel, and one took almost eight months. And well worth the time.

But wait! When my horse's shoe falls off, he starts limping almost immediately. And when the shoe is nailed back on, suddenly he's fine. Doesn't hurt anymore. Proof that the shoe is better for him than barefoot.

Have you ever crossed your legs for so long that your foot goes to sleep? We all have, and we all know what's happening. The leg-cross has cut off the circulation to the foot, and with no circulation, the nerve endings lose their sensitivity and fail to work. The second you uncross, or stand up, the circulation returns, as do the nerve endings.

Ooohh! Ouch!

The same thing happens to a horse when a metal shoe is nailed on. The inability of the hoof to flex removes its ability to pump blood, virtually eliminating circulation in the hoof mechanism. Without proper circulation, the nerve endings quit transmitting, and the horse no longer feels the "ouch." When the shoe falls off, the circulation returns and suddenly he can feel again.

Whoa, what's that about??

Convince yourself. Try this test. On a cool day, or under cover, feel the hoof and lower leg of a shod horse, and a hoof of another who is barefoot. The barefoot horse's lower leg and hoof will feel warm to the touch, because of the blood circulating within. The shod horse's lower leg and hoof will be cool, not warm, because of the blood that is not circulating within.

As mentioned earlier, our Scribbles took a good seven to eight months to regain a healthy hoof with no ouch. And today he's a happy camper, on asphalt or concrete, on the trail, in the arena. His hooves are beautifully concaved, keeping the coffin bone up where it belongs. They are beveled at the edges, just like a wild horse's hoof. And they're as hard as stone.

The sacrifice? The downside?

A few months time to let him grow the hoof nature always intended for him to have. Good boy, Scribbles.

How much trimming is needed, and how often, depends upon the horse's environment and lifestyle. Remember, the objective is to help the horse replicate the hoof that he would grow if he were living in the wild, moving eight to twenty miles a day with the herd. If he's living in a Virginia pasture or, heaven forbid, a box stall and not moving around much, there will be a lot more trimming, probably more often, than if he were living in a high desert natural "pasture" like we had in California and moving around all day wearing down his own hooves. But the objective can be reached in any case.

Pete Ramey, a hoof specialist who teaches hoof care all over the world, believes we have only just begun to discover the true potential of the wild horse model. After a trip to wild horse country for research he said, "The country was solid rock; mostly baseball-sized porous volcanic rock that you could literally use as a rasp to work a hoof if you wanted to. Horse tracks were fairly rare, because there was so little dirt between the rocks. There were a few muddy areas from the recent snow melt, but they were littered with rocks as well. The horses made no attempt to find these softer spots to walk on."

Pete and his wife, Ivy, observed, videotaped, and photographed at least sixty horses. All of them, from the foals to the aged, moved effortlessly and efficiently across the unbelievably harsh terrain. According to Pete, the horses were doing collected, extended trots across an obstacle course that would shame the best show ring work of any dressage horse, with their tails high in the air and their heads cocked over their shoulders watching the intruding couple.

"I have never known a horse I would attempt to ride in this terrain," Pete says. "Ivy and I had to literally watch our every step when we were walking. The movement of the horses was not affected by the slippery dusting of snow on the rocks. In fact, they got around much better than the mule deer and the pronghorns. The entire time we were there we did not see a limp, or even a 'give' to any rock, or a single lame horse, and not one chip or split in any of their hooves. It was an unbelievable sight."

The world has been shocked and amazed by the ability of Pete and others to forge rock-crushing bare hooves, boost equine performance, and treat "incurable" hoof disease. "I don't want to diminish these facts," Pete says, "but I now realize that we haven't even scratched the tip of the iceberg."

Pete is my hero! He is much of the reason for the existence of my book *The Soul of Horse*. He cares so very much about the horse and proves it daily by how much time he spends researching the complex internal workings of the horse's hoof and the myriad factors that affect its health. And substantiating that research on the horses in his care. In his DVD series, *Under the Horse*, Pete lays every bit of it out for us. If you've ever doubted the fact that horses do not need metal shoes and are in fact better off without them, please see this series.

Pete will convince you of this undeniable truth. In my humble belief, whether or not you ever intend to trim your own horse's feet, *Under the Horse* is one of the most valuable and user-friendly compilations of knowledge, research, and insight for improving the health and lifespan of your horse that exists on the planet. And believe it or not, The American Farriers Association (the metal shoe group) agrees. An excerpt from their review:

"Pete Ramey's set of DVD's is without a doubt a must-have series for any equine professional farrier or horse owner. Pete Ramey offers wisdom and insight that his years of practice and study have given him. If you own only one hoof care DVD series, this should be it." American Farriers Journal

Pretty impressive for an organization of metal shoers.

There's an old expression: No hoof, no horse. And the reams of research I've pored over truly made that point. So much of what can go wrong with a horse begins or is controlled by the health of the hoof. When that hoof is healthy, is flexing, and taking stress off the heart, it can add years to a horse's life.

And he'll be happier.

Not only because he feels better, but because he can actually feel the surface he's walking on, which makes him more comfortable and more secure in his footing. It's the way nature intended. Would you run on the beach with boots on? Or do you want to feel the sand between your toes? Not a perfect analogy, but you get the idea (See Happier Healthier Horses).

The president of the American Farrier's Association, in a speech to his constituency reported in the organization's publication, said that 95% of all the domestic horses on this planet have some degree of lameness. I wonder if he told them why. Or that hoof lameness simply does not happen in the wild. Dr. Jay Kirkpatrick, director of the Science and Conservation Center in Billings, Montana, has studied wild horses most of his adult life and says that lameness in the wild is extremely rare and virtually every case he's seen is related to arthritic shoulder joints, not hoof problems.

All of the above is why our horses' shoes came off. How could I know all this, understand all this, and not do it. I had, after all, promised Cash.

So think about it. Think seriously about it every time you hear someone say that what they do for a living is better for your horse than what the horse would do for itself in the wild. Ponder the presidents of those tobacco companies testifying before Congress, emphatic that tobacco was not harmful. Dig around on your own. Do some research. Compare what "the experts" say. Gather your own knowledge and don't let someone else make decisions for you. Whether it's about your horses, or your life.

And if you do own a horse, show him that he's not an ox, or a tractor, or a motorcycle. He's your partner.

And let him know by your leadership that you love him and will give him the best care you possibly can.

5

RAISON D'ETRE

Every horse on the planet is born to be wild.

This has all been discussed before, but some of it bears repeating.

Domestic horses and wild horses are genetically exactly the same. That means that the horse living in your back yard or at a stable somewhere is genetically the same as the horse who evolved in the wild and those still living in the wild. The belief of some that a few hundred years of selective breeding can change all that is scientifically impossible because it takes between 5000 and 10,000 years to even begin to change the base genetics of any species.

Which means the horses in our back yard have been programmed for millions and millions of years to live in wide open spaces where they can see predators coming, eat small bits of grass forage around the clock up to 18 to 20 hours a day, move 8-20 miles a day, on bare feet that can flex with each step to circulate blood within the hoof capsules, live with multiple horses for safety and security, and even balance their own diets if provided with enough choices to do so.

I had to smile at Cash a few months back. I was just sitting in the Gator way up the hill gawking at the herd after distributing half a bale of Bermuda hay in the western pasture. We still do this even in the Spring and Summer to help ensure maximum movement for the horses and to give them an additional way to balance the high sugars of the cool season grasses that pop up in the early Spring before the creeping tentacles of the Bermuda (warm season grass, low sugar) come alive. It's always interesting to me that even with all the sweet Spring grasses around – and clover, oh my gosh clover is everywhere! – they still usually race to the hay when I put it out. I had a foot propped up on the dash of the Gator, just taking it all in, hoping perhaps for a fecal sample from Noelle, when I heard something behind me. It was Cash, very close, nibbling away at blades of grass, not hay. I dialed in the focus to see if he was eating the same grass each bite or having himself a varied diet. When we moved from southern California we were warned by many that horses could not be out 24/7 on the rich grasses of middle Tennessee. That made no sense to me so I started researching. Went straightaway to wild horses for my lessons. I discovered that the pasture the horse needs isn't pretty. Not what you'd expect to see driving through Kentucky, or even our little slice of middle Tennessee. So our pasture is ugly with a capital "U".

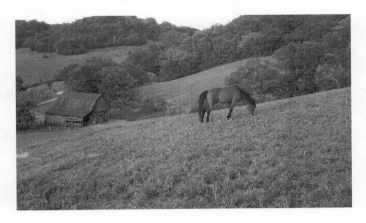

Seven or eight different kinds of native grasses (none genetically modified), lots of weeds, berries, brambles, bushes, and trees of all kinds. Choices. Lots of them. Most of the horse pastures around here are thick carpets of a single type of cool season grass (high sugar) without a weed or a tree, chemically fertilized and sprayed for pests and weeds. All bad for the horse. If you give a horse no choice, he'll eat whatever's there to stay alive. Give him all the choices he needs and he'll take better care of himself than we humans can.

Because, of course, Mr. Cash's genetics are identical to those of the horses in the wild, all of whom have evolved over millions and millions of years and thanks to God and Mother Nature they know how to take care of themselves with no help from us humans. If they didn't, we would've never known the horse. He'd be extinct. My Cash could be turned loose into the wild where there are other horses and he would be just fine.

Not happening of course! But he would figure it out. As would any domestic horse. So the problem is not in the horse's genetics but with us humans who cannot, as Rick Lamb says, "Set them up for success and then get the heck outta the way."

Cash was browsing along using his nose, lips, and even his tongue to distinguish one blade from another. It was fascinating to watch. He was very picky and mowing almost faster than I could watch. The way he was using his tongue was so intriguing it was difficult to focus on which blade of grass was disappearing. But focus I did and was pleased that he was rejecting the clover. How many times had I been told to keep clover out of a pasture at all costs? Too much sugar! Cash would take a bit of fescue, a bite of orchard, balance it with some (warm season, low sugar) crab-like grass, an undistinguished weed here and there, but never a bite of clover. Not one. Once he even nuzzled into a big patch of clover and I thought *Aha!* But he was only after a couple of blades of grass hidden right square in the middle of the clover. Not one shamrock passed between his teeth. Then he met up with the long string of hay stretching out toward the west and settled in with the others making pilgrimage toward the setting sun.

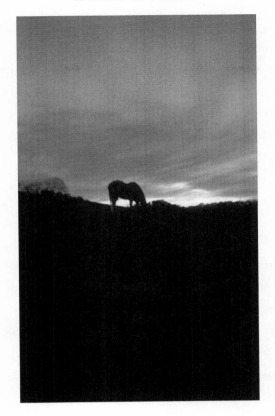

Choices, I thought. The wild horses had assured me that if I give our guys and gals all the choices they need or want they will take care of themselves. A horse's genetics know what the horse needs and when. If a horse needs a liver cleansing the brain will send him after thistle. When he needs vitamin E it might send him searching for a blackberry. Etc. If he's eaten quite enough of high-sugar grasses, he'll switch to the low sugar grasses to balance. When humans attempt to perform these functions, it's usually pure guesswork, and usually late, behind the curve.

I knew all this from the research but I must admit it was quite exhilarating to see it in play right in front of my eyes. I just sat there watching these happy magnificent creatures until the sun finally disappeared behind the hill, feeling very good about the choices we made so our herd would have the choices they needed.

It seems that word, *choice*, has come up again and again as we've made our way through this relatively new journey with horses. We started there actually by learning to give the horse the choice whether or not to be in relationship with us. And the choice of how they would prefer to be trained, to work together.

Our herd has been out 24/7 for almost seven years at this writing. Half of it in the arid, grass-less high desert of southern California and half in the wet, lush, loaded-with-grass of middle Tennessee.

Back in the beginning our herd all lived in a manner diametrically opposed to what their genetics were calling for. They were cooped up in tiny little stalls where they could move, by actual count, an average of only 800 steps in a 24-hour day as opposed to the 8-20 miles a day their genetics called for. And we ultimately discovered that such a huge differential was not just affecting physical structure, it was affecting their digestion, their breathing, the health of their feet, and thereby immensely affecting their stress levels. This virtual continuous movement when horses are out, we've learned recently, is likely to be one of the most important pieces to the entire jigsaw puzzle.

And, as mentioned above, horses are genetically programmed to eat grass forage (real grass or grass hay), little bits at a time, up to 18-20 hours a day. Free-choice. Around the clock.

And we discovered that a horse in a stall who cannot commune with other horses gains yet another level of stress to endure. The purpose of the herd for a prey animal is safety and security. Being with other like animals is quite literally a safety net. There are more eyes to see trouble coming. Being deprived of that comfort, at some level, breeds huge amounts of stress.

But as I mentioned earlier, we knew none of this fewer than seven years ago when we made the big leap into horses without a single clue. Maybe it helped, as they say, to come in with a clean plate. No baggage. No knowledge. Just an obsessive and compulsive urge to offer our new family members the very best life that we could. That urge-turned-insane-quest not only culminated in our herd living a life very close to the one they were genetically programmed to live, it spawned our first two books, *The Soul of a Horse – Life Lessons from the Herd*, a best seller thank you so much, and *The Soul of a Horse Blogged – The Journey Continues*, which together have changed the lives of thousands of horses and people all across the planet (see *Happier Healthier*

Horses Around the World on our website), for which Kathleen and I will be eternally grateful. Thankfully they are also humorous books. When you start where we started and really push the envelope there's going to be a lot of stumbling around, a bunch of wrong turns, botched efforts, and, yes, stooopid mistakes. But, the trip has been so worth it and we are ever grateful to God for the opportunity to help make this planet a little better than we found it.

Which is why we needed to know all this. Our horses were born to be wild and we needed to know why. And what we should do about it. Cash, Mouse, Noelle, Mariah, Pocket, Saffron, Firestorm, and Skeeter tell us how grateful they are everyday of our lives, and I can promise you there is no better feeling on earth.

6

Bon Appetit

Why is the subject of feeding your horse so complex? Or why is it made to *seem* so complex? It could be that too many humans are trying to figure out what *they* think the horse needs, instead of just asking the horse. And there's the issue of convenience. What's easy. Either for the owner or the barn manager who has perhaps dozens of horses to look after. And then trying to fix the problems caused by following such a doctrine. Or cover up the problems. Not unlike taking a Tylenol for a headache. Instead of attacking the cause of the headache we cover it up. Make it seem like it's not there.

Let's say the headache is caused by stress. Get rid of the stress and you not only eliminate the headache you probably solve a whole tub full of other problems at the same time.

But is it likely that we will do that?

Probably not.

We're human. We can think and rationalize on many levels. We have work stress, relationship stress, money stress, kid stress, whatever.

And we inflict all of that on ourselves by the choices we make.

The horse doesn't do that. He doesn't make those choices and does not inflict the outcome of bad choices upon himself.

If a horse is stressed the source of that stress does not come from the horse. Or from another horse. Think about it. This is a prey animal, a flight animal, who is genetically designed to live outdoors, in a herd, with lots of room where he can see what's coming from every direction, while collecting ten to twenty miles of movement every day of his life.

So what do you figure happens to him when he is made to live in a 12x12 stall, inside some structure, with no movement whatsoever, and no herd for safety; where he cannot see a predator coming after him from over the hill?

Stress.

Big time.

Ever wonder why a horse starts cribbing?

Spend a day, a full 24-hour day, in a horse stall in some barn.

Seriously. Do it. Without any other humans around. No one to talk to.

See how crazed you are after that experience. And you aren't even a prey animal. You're a predator. You're supposed to *like* small cozy caves.

Horses don't.

And your body doesn't need to move continually, virtually around the clock, to keep itself working as its supposed to work. You might be better off if you *did* walk all those miles, but its' not necessary for function. With horses it is. And you don't *need* other humans to feel safe and secure. Horses *need* other horses.

So what happens when that stress bubbles up and he starts cribbing? The humans put a "miracle" cribbing collar on him, or a muzzle, and/or paint the stall with some bitter solution, feed him various mineral mixes, or – yes, they're available – put an electrical shock collar on him. All when there is a very simple solution to the problem. Eliminate the source of the stress. Get the horse out of that stall.

Have you ever heard of a wild horse cribbing? Or a domestic horse who is outside moving 24/7? I haven't.

As mentioned earlier, a horse in a stall will move, on average, only 800 steps in a 24-hour day. When every part of his body is genetically programmed to move 10 to 20 miles in that same 24 hour period. That movement is continually flexing his bare hooves which generates a massive amount of blood circulation, both in the hoof and up the leg, taking a substantial load off the heart. His movement not only assists digestion it's *necessary* for *proper* digestion. And it keeps his muscles toned, and eliminates boredom, stress, and quite frankly makes him happy.

So what does any of this have to do with diet and nutrition?

Everything. Because the horse's health and happiness is a jigsaw puzzle of closely interlocking pieces.

We continue to learn every day about how we can ensure that our horses are getting, or have access to, the kind of options they would have available to them in the wild, which is the foundation for their genetic structure – and our approach to everything equine – to ensure that our horses have access to what they **need**, and, at least to some extent, can also pick and choose what **they feel** they need based upon their individual conditions. As is highlighted throughout our books and website, for us, it's not about what we humans think, or what is most convenient for us. It's about how we can replicate as closely as possible the health and happiness our horses would have if they were in the wild taking care of themselves. I feel we are now giant steps closer to my goal of seeing our horses live happily and healthily into their thirties and forties.

When we first got into horses, I researched, searched, dug, and asked *whyyyy* for months before ultimately came up with the following specifics:

1. Feed free-choice grass hay around the clock.

This is a must because, in the wild, horses are moving and eating up to 18 to 20 hours a day. Their tiny tummies (comparatively speaking) need to be eating little bits of grass or grass hay pretty much *all* the time. Horses are genetically programmed to eat grass forage (real grass or grass hay), little bits at a time, up to 18-20

hours a day. The horse's stomach is programmed to release digestive acid around the clock. Acid that digests
grass (not sugar, not alfalfa, not pellets, not carrots, just
grass or grass hay). When that grass forage is not dribbling into the hind gut on a regular basis the acid has
nothing to work on but the insides of the horse itself!
Unlike humans whose digestive acid turns on and off
depending upon whether food is present, the horse's
digestive acid never stops. So the grass forage needs to
be there. Free-choice. Around the clock.

The problem is that even the best farm-grown,
grass hay, although necessary, will not give your horse
all the choices he needs to get the vitamins, minerals,
and nutrients he needs and can acquire on his own in
the wild, because it's only *one* kind of hay. In the wild
the horse eats multiple kinds of grasses and myriad
brambles, trees, bushes, etc. And in the wild, what he's
eating has not been fertilized to beat the band and
grown and regrown on the same soil each year. If we
could feed three or four *different* types of grass hay (alfalfa is *not* a grass hay) every day, we could give the
horses at least a few choices and get much closer to the
mixture horses have access to in the wild, but many of
us can't afford the time, effort, and cost of doing that so
we resort to supplements to attempt to fill in the gaps.
A single kind of grass or grass hay will simply not be
offering all the vitamins, nutrients, minerals, antioxi-

dants, and EFAs (the omegas 3,6 & 9) that a horse could scrounge for itself in the wild.

2. Feed a "condiment-sized" serving of alfalfa

Lisa Ross-Williams says think of alfalfa as a condiment, like salt, pepper, hot sauce, or salad dressing. Just a taste, for the variety, protein, and different nutrients. Only a taste because alfalfa is way higher in calcium than your horse needs and the calcium/phosphorous ratio is way out of whack. It's even worse in the southwest quadrant of the United States because of the high alkalinity of the soil. I have a stone the size of a cantaloupe that Dr. Matt removed from a horse who was being fed 100% alfalfa. It's a terrific reminder to keep alfalfa in small portions. In California, our boys and girls got a total of three small flakes a day divided among five horses, scattered in maybe ten small piles, morning and evening, so everybody was assured of getting their fair share. Here in middle Tennessee their very natural pasture contains at least five different grasses plus weeds, brambles, trees, clover, dandelions, etc. etc. and they receive no alfalfa at all.

3. We were also told to feed a half scoop of Strategy for each horse, morning and evening. We did for a while... but not anymore.

This was the vet's way of adding nutrients, minerals, and vitamins to the diet, but ultimately, as I dug deeper, it became apparent that this was not the best way because I have found that virtually all pelleted "total feeds" have things in them that horses would never have in the wild and *shouldn't* have (based upon all the reading I've done) in their domestic feed. Every natural "expert" I've read agrees that a horse's total sugar intake (NSC, which means non-structured carbohydrate) should be 10% or less of his entire intake. Hay or feed that is higher than 10% sugar is setting your horse up for all sorts of potential problems. Oats and corn, once in the body, are very much like eating pure sugar. And molasses *is* pure sugar. Just Google "NSC Horse Feeds" and you'll find plenty to read on the subject. I found a list of the NSC levels in various Purina Feeds and it was scary. I prefer not to publish the entire list here because hopefully Purina is continuously working to bring their NSC numbers down. Suffice to say Omolene 100 was over 40% NSC at this writing. Strategy was 26%. And only two out of 16 feeds on the list were 10%.

Note:
Triple Crown Lite NSC is 10%
Triple Crown Safe Starch Forage (which is what we use) is guaranteed to be *less* than 10%
    All grain is exceedingly high in glycemic index.
Here are a few:
Corn – 117
Oats – 100
Wheat 71
Carrots 51

Whereas Bermuda grass hay has a glycemic index of 23, and rice bran 22. On the Glycemic scale these are low. I've tried for years to find a "rule of thumb" calculator for conversion of Glycemic Index to NSC, and vice versa. But have never found such an animal because whereas both measurements relate to sugar content, they measure different things. I do know that Bermuda hay is "generally" in the 7% to 9% range NSC. It can be lower or higher depending upon when it's cut, where it's grown, etc, etc. But generally speaking Bermuda, a warm season grass, is much lower in NSC than cool season grasses like Orchard, Timothy, or Fescue (see our books: *Horses Were Born to Be On Grass* and *Horses Without Grass* and *The Soul of a Horse Blogged – The Journey Continues*).

If the ratio of Bermuda at say 8% NSC roughly equals a Glycemic Index of 23, that would mean the Glycemic Index is almost three times the NSC number.

If that ratio holds up and down the ladder (and I have no information that says whether it truly does or doesn't), then oats would have an NSC of about 32 (quite high), and corn would have an NSC of 39. Corn and Oats are in virtually every bagged, pelleted feed available for horses.

Then there is the issue of processed fats, which in a bag of feed must be processed to keep the fats from going rancid... BUT the processing, heat processing and hydrogenation, mutates the fat causing all sorts of free radicals in the body, in effect "rusting" our horse's veins as Dr. Dan, the natural horse vet puts it. Those same mutated fats "rust" *our* veins as well, which is why neither our horses nor ourselves should eat processed fats. Fats, themselves, are not bad. In fact they're good. It's what the manufacturer does to them to "stabilize" them that is bad for our health. Kathleen and I stick to cold-pressed extra virgin olive oil, coconut oil, and peanut oil.

So, when I finally decided it was time to bite the bullet, to start digging into nutrition, there we were, with our horses quite used to getting a treat every morning (the molasses/grain based Strategy at 26% NSC) in order to intake some of the vitamins/minerals/nutrients not found in their farm-grown hay. These vitamins/minerals/nutrients are all available as supplements, but how were we to get these supplements down the horses (most of the supplements available for purchase are in powder or granular form) without something to mix them with, something these powders will stick to and thus wind up willingly going down the gullets of our horses... without a bunch of NSCs and processed fats going down as well. This was my problem, and my search, for quite some time. Grains won't work. Too much sugar. And every processed feed I've found is either based heavily on grains, or has processed fats, or molasses, or all of the above.

But at last, I found it. A feed called Safe Starch from Triple Crown.

Safe Starch is a complete feed. But it's not a pellet, and has no grains or molasses, and is guaranteed to be under the safe recommended 10% NSC (sugar). It's a "chopped forage" in a bag. We call it chopped salad. At first I was put off... too bulky... weird looking... and... well, not a pellet. But I finally opened the bag and tried it. A full scoop, loose, not packed, weighs only 13+ ounces. So even though it's a complete balanced feed, it can also be a great base, or "carrier" for powdered supplements, which is what I'd been looking for. And the horse isn't eating pellets, he's eating what he's supposed to be eating! Grass forage. The main base is chopped Orchard and Timothy hay, held loosely together with a touch of Soybean oil, and mixed with a vitamin/mineral premix and Triple Crown's Equimix nutrients. All guaranteed less than 10% NSC. Yes, that soybean oil is processed but I look at it this way: This is the best there is on the feed-in-a-bag world. Or at least the best I've ever found after extensive search. There is no sugar and no grain. Just grass hay which the horse should be consuming around the clock anyway. Triple Crown actually started out with a cold-processed oil but there just wasn't enough shelf life (leave olive oil out on a piece of bread for a couple of months and take a sniff). And there is very minimal oil, especially in the less-than-

two-scoops a day our horses get. So we use it exclusive-
ly.

It's the best alternative I've seen. It's real grass hay,
thus the proper kind of chewing/roughage/etc... plus it
contains all the stuff the horses would be nibbling for
themselves if in the wild.

And for those of us who only want a small amount
to use as a safe "carrier" to serve as an "appetizer" over
which to sprinkle vitamins, Omega 3s, antioxidants and
the like, it seems to me to be a terrific choice. The only
choice really. No sugars, grains, or molasses. Only a bit
of Soybean oil, any mutating of which can be countered
with a good Omega 3 supplement, and/or a good anti-
oxidant like grapeseed extract, or vitamin E, etc. And
we can continue with whatever supplements we like the
best for each of our boys and girls because, at less than a
pound in the morning and evening, they aren't getting
enough of Triple Crown's vitamin/mineral/etc to cause
any concern or conflict with the supplements I prefer to
tailor for each of our horses.

And all eight of ours like it! We transitioned completely from Strategy pellets, and all of our horses are
making happy plates, leaving nothing in their tubs.
Yippee!

The recommended Safe Starch serving for a 1000
pound horse (as a complete feed) is between 10 to 20
pounds a day, with the norm being on the mid-high
side of that "to keep horses in good shape." So, figure

15 pounds as the average recommended serving per day (18-20 full scoops) if using as a complete feed. But, again, we are using approximately a scoop a day depending upon the supplements each horse gets, morning and night, so it's approximately 8% of the vitamin/mineral mix the manufacturer recommends if using as a complete feed; so I'm not at all concerned about over-dosing the vitamins/minerals/ etc. when my stuff is added. Only our old guy Skeeter, and young Miss Mouse get a bit more, with a some rice bran added (depending upon the time of year – see the book *Horses Were Born to be on Grass*).

For the exact amounts of what we feed morning and evening please see the diet page of our website, as it does tend to vary from time to time as we become better informed.

One last emphasis: Emerging research regarding fat in a horse's diet is paralleling the studies for humans with similar results. Fat is necessary for both of us... **but only if it's unrefined, unprocessed, unhydrogenated** fat. It's the processing that manufacturers do to "preserve" the fat that is killing us and our horses, the heat-processed, chemically-mutated fat. I heard a worthy phrase recently: *Eat sugar and you'll burn sugar and store fat (*in other words: *get* fat.*)* But if you *Eat fat you will burn fat.* There are good articles on this subject all over the internet. Google is good.

7

THE BOND

Dr. Marty Becker says in his wonderful book *The Healing Power of Pets*, "We should recognize the bond for what it is — living proof of the powerful connectedness between mankind and the rest of the animal kingdom. And the element of this powerful relationship that has always impressed me the most was the importance of nurturing another creature."

I wonder if those who don't believe that you can bond with a horse, also dismiss Dr. Becker's statement about the importance of nurturing another creature.

Not long ago I was hauling my tripod and video camera down our very steep pasture, struggling a bit because of sore ribs, a remnant from my fall off a ladder. I was moaning to myself about it as I set up the camera to videotape herd movement. Five of our six horses would soon begin their meandering climb back up the steep grade toward where the camera was set up. Only Mariah had remained at the top.

After a moment, I heard her shuffling up behind me. She paused at my back, lip-nibbled my shirtsleeve, then the most amazing thing happened. She nudged her nose between my arm and my ribs and pressed her warm muzzle softly against my rib cage. Precisely where it was hurting. She didn't move for minutes, until I had to shift position to start taping. It was a moment I didn't want to end.

How did she know?

Moreover, why did she care?

This is the horse whose relationship with humans was a blank stare when we first met her.

This is the bond.

Cash and Mariah are both what I call mutt Arabs (un-papered). They hang out a lot together. Not always, but I would say that they spend more time near each other than with any other horse in the herd. But that's it. No hugging and kissing. Not even any swapped grooming that I've ever seen. Yet, when Mariah broke the ice in our pond and fell in she managed to get out on her own and make it back to the front paddock of the barn. (see her chapter in *The Soul of a Horse Blogged – The Journey Continues*). When I found her, Cash was next to her pressing his body into hers, clearly trying to give her needed warmth. I never before or since have seen them that close together. Cash was there when she needed him.

Just as Mariah was there when I needed her.

But we must not only savor those moments. We must understand them from the perspective of the horse and not try to force our humanness on them.

Kathleen and I spend regular time in the pasture, without agenda, to foster this bond. And to learn about our horses. The relationship, generated originally with Join-Up, or our No Agenda Time, or other methods, always gives the horse the choice of whether or not to be with us. We do not force relationship on them. They choose it. And it continues to mature because of our time in the pasture. And we become better communicators. Everything about the relationship gets better.

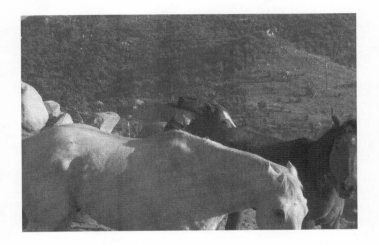

Time in the saddle, in the arena, and on the trail are important. But I believe the most important time is in the pasture. Just hanging out. It has done wonders for us, and our horses.

It continually strengthens the bond, and our relationship.

It teaches us about the horse, his habits, his language, his individual personality, and his genetics. How to read and understand what makes him tick.

It strengthens our leadership, and the horse's respect.

It dispels fear, both ours and theirs.

It breeds confidence.

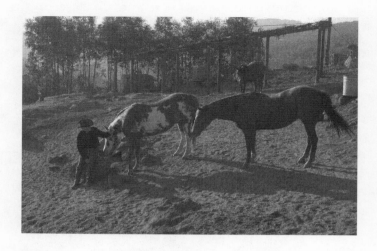

And it eliminates stress because they never ever worry about whether something bad will be afoot when we're around.

None of that can be injected, like a flu shot. It doesn't come as a flash when we wake up one morning, no matter how much we wish that it would. And even though books and DVDs have certainly crammed us full of insight and knowledge, they cannot replace the benefits of experience that come with being there, doing it, absorbing, learning firsthand.

Mileage.

And proving to them, just as with other humans, that you will first speak their language before asking them to learn yours. That you will do something they feel is worthwhile, before asking them to believe that what you want is worthwhile.

Spending time with the horses, learning from their end of the lead rope, also reminds us to always be thinking ahead, questioning, anticipating what could happen or go wrong by doing things this way or that.

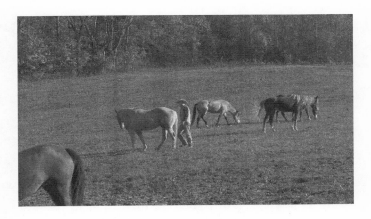

Our time in the pasture, observing, studying, interacting at the horse's discretion, has taught us so much. That's why we wouldn't pay someone else to do the morning and evening feeding, even if our budget could afford it. Yes, there are mornings when we'd love to sleep in. But doing our own feeding guarantees no less than a couple of hours a day with our horses. Over time, those hours help to dissect and internalize each horse's individual personality, which determines how leadership is expressed in different ways to different horses. It provides insight into how weather affects their behavior. It has taught us, virtually by osmosis, how subtle our language can be, or not, with each unique horse. And it continually confirms us as members of the herd.

"I just never have enough time," one woman said to me.

"Then maybe you should acquire something that doesn't depend upon your leadership, relationship, compassion, and understanding for its health and happiness."

I didn't really say that, but I *thought* it. Under Kathleen's guidance I *am* learning :).

Why, I wonder, are we still where we are today, with so many owners of horses missing the very best part of horse ownership? The reason, I believe, is that most people do not begin at the beginning. They want to start halfway around the track, instead of in the starting gate.

I now have a horse. I want to do something with it. Go riding. Compete. Something!

We humans are in such a hurry that there's no time to build a relationship. To learn to communicate. To gain and give understanding. To walk in the horse's boots, so to speak.

To begin at the beginning.

The beginning for us was building relationship through our discovery of Monty Roberts and his Join-Up process.

Why?

I ask that question a lot.

To a fault.

Kathleen says it often seems that *why* is the only word I know.

Whyyyy?

So, *why* do I feel so strongly about *Monty Roberts' Join-Up?* Or *No Agenda Time*, our version of Join Up without a round pen?

Because they answer the *why* questions right up front:

Why does this work?

Because it speaks to the horse's genetics in the horse's own language, the language of the herd. Which is all built upon the fact that the horse is a prey animal, a flight animal. And safety and security are his number one concern, at the top of his forever wish list. The horse would always rather be in a safe and secure, stress free relationship than not.

Why do you say anyone can do Join Up? Or No Agenda Time?

Because they are simple. Easy to accomplish. Straight to the point. Join Up uses a very specific "1-2-3" kind of "to-do" list that anyone can understand and handle. I managed to accomplish Join-Up after watching Monty's DVD only twice (previous chapter).

And No Agenda Time (link in the resource section of this book) uses virtually nothing other than your will power to keep your hands and brain to yourself.

Why does it cause the horse to – as you say – change forever?

Because, in either method, the horse does the joining-up of his own free will. He chooses you, not vice-versa. It's his choice whether or not to say to you *I trust you to be my leader.* If you in any way coerce the horse into being close to you, into accepting you or your training, there will be no change in the horse. The willingness, the "try" will not be there.

But... once the Join-Up has been accomplished of the horse's choice, continuing to be a good leader is the number one goal. The determining factor of who *leads* who in the herd is who *moves* who. That means ground work on your part, and lots of it. And this is where a lot of folks get into trouble and don't understand the outcome.

Many like to think that once Joined-Up the horse is going to be like a smoochie puppy. It's all going to be cuddles and hugs and kisses. But a horse is not a smoochie puppy, not even close. The horse's idea of a good relationship, first and foremost, is a feeling of safety. The security of knowing he is being lead by a good leader who will keep him safe. The horse doesn't fall in love with the horse above him in the herd, or out of love with the one below him. And this is difficult for most humans to grasp. They want relationship to be an emotional thing, but it simply isn't in the life and language of the herd. Yes, they can like being with you, but mostly it's about security.

Not to say that once the horse's security, his trust, is well in place there won't be a bond. There will be. Very much so. It'll just be different than what most humans perceive as a bond. There could even be a shared hug or kiss here and there with some horses, but not necessarily with all horses. It depends upon the personality of the horse. We have eight and they're all different. Some show moments of affection, some not so much. But the bond and relationship is strong with all of them.

And because of Join-up they all give back, try harder, and are more willing. And they all feel safe and comfortable when with Kathleen or myself.

What your relationship turns into after Join-Up depends upon you and how good a leader you are. In other words, how well and how easily you can move the horse's every-body-part whenever and wherever you want. Another concept that is sometimes hard for humans to grasp: the simple idea that who moves who can determine leadership, bolster relationship, and select one's place in the herd.

But, as mentioned above, Monty's Join-Up in a round pen is not the only way to begin a relationship with your horse? There are more ways to Join Up than one can count.

Our Mouse had not been exposed to the round pen join-up when she made her choice to Join Up. It all happened with Monty in a "square pen". Back in Iowa it took six men to get Mouse into a trailer to come to Monty. It took Monty ten minutes to convince her, using her language, to come to him and say *I trust you to be my leader.* A moment later Monty was addressing his group of students using Mouse's back as a podium to lean on. Just amazing.

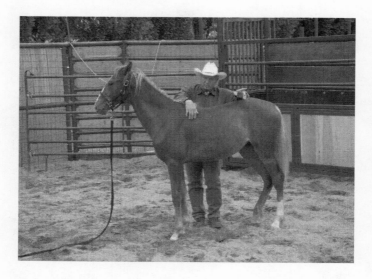

Saffron, our new mustang who came to us pregnant, from the wild via the BLM, made her choice on the evening of my birthday as Kathleen and I sat in her paddock during our regular No-Agenda Time. Like a switch was thrown. From zero to a hundred in an instant. See our blog post: *An Amazing Birthday Gift from a Wild Mustang.*

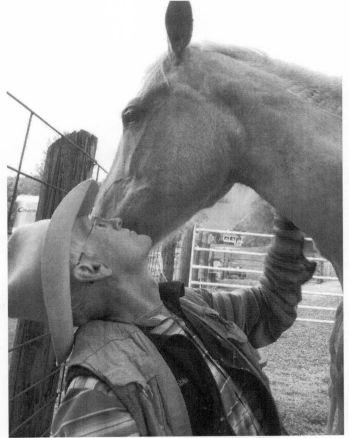

Saffron made her choice on my birthday

But every version of Join Up that truly works depends upon those two key ingredients that must be present or the relationship will never be what it should be, what it could be.

It must be the horse's choice to trust you or not, to be in relationship with you, or not. And you must continue prove to the horse that you are his leader, a *good* leader. In *his* language. Those two ingredients are Monty's secret ingredients. No one else, in my experience, has ever made it as clear or as simple as Monty.

Pat and Linda Parelli have their own way of accomplishing the same end relationship with their horses, which definitely includes giving the horse the choice to trust and be in relationship. They just don't call it join-up and it's not as simple or as "1-2-3" as Monty's Join-Up.

The bottom line is that after we put in the time and effort, when we got the relationship and leadership right, when we did it from the horse's end of the lead rope, not our own, our horses changed.

Every one of them.

Each differently perhaps, but change they did.

And always for the better.

Like Cash in the beginning, the others have never stopped trying, never stopped listening, never stopped giving.

Why would we do it any other way?

8

CARPE DIEM

Early on in this amazing journey with horses we spent an incredible amount of time out in the pasture. In the round pen. Feeding. And just hanging out. Observing. Listening. Learning. It's amazing what you'll hear when you listen. Here's how my Cash put it in the Introduction to *The Soul of a Horse – Life Lessons from the Herd:*

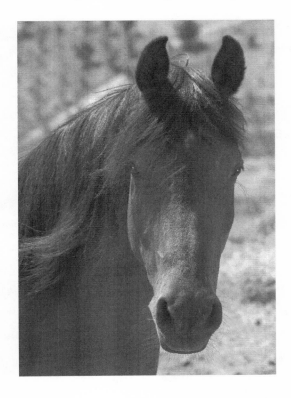

My name is Cash. I am horse. I have been on this planet for some fifty-two million years. Well, not me personally. My ancestors. It all began in North America, somewhere near what is now called Utah. We hung out and evolved for most of that time, then we began to migrate to South America, and across the Bering Straits Bridge to Asia, Europe, and Africa. And, eventually, some ten thousand years after we left, we were brought back home by the Spanish conquistadors.

We've been through it all. Ice Ages. Volcanic periods. Meteor strikes. Dinosaurs. You name it. And we survived.

We've only been carrying man around for, oh, the last three to four thousand years. We've helped him farm, hunt, travel, and fight his enemies. We were helping man shape world history, winning wars for him, as far back as 1345 BC. We protected kings' dominions in medieval times, carried knights into the Crusades, fought on European battlefields all the way into the early 1900s, and we helped conquer and settle the American West.

Throughout these millions of years, many of us have remained wild and free. Even today, our herds roam free in Australia, New Zealand, Mongolia, France, Africa, the Greek Island of Cephalonia, Abaco in the Bahamas, Sable Island in Nova Scotia, the Canadian West, several states of the American West, Virginia, and North Carolina.

And until recently, we've done it all pretty much naked and in good relationship with man. But over the past several hundred years things began to change. Changes that are actually inexplicable, given that our genetics and history are widely known. You see, we are not cave dwellers. We don't like dark cozy rooms, clothing, iron shoes, heat, air conditioning, and we're not built to stand around all day in one place eating from a tub virtually withers high.

Humans seem to like all that. And because they do they presume we should like it too. But we're movers and shakers. In the wild we'll move ten to twenty miles a day, keeping our hooves flexing and circulating blood, feeding our tiny little stomachs a little at a time, and keeping our own thermoregulatory systems in good working order.

Think about it. Our survival through all those millions of years has built a pretty darned determined genetic system. And an excellent formula for survival. We are what you humans call prey animals, flight animals. We are not predators, like you. We have survived because we freak out at every little thing, race off and don't look back. We are also herd animals. Not just because it's fun to be around our pals, but because there is safety in numbers. And being a prey animal, safety is just about the most important thing to us. But our idea of safety is not the same as yours. Our genetic history does not understand being all alone in a twelve-by-twelve stall. Even if it's lined in velvet, in a heated barn, it's away from the herd and by no stretch of the emotion or imagination is that a safe haven! Stress is all we get from such an experience.

Stress. Big time!

Have you ever seen one of us, locked in a stall, pacing... pawing... swaying... gnawing? That horse is saying Let me outta here!! I need to move! I need to circulate some blood!

And about these metal shoes nailed to our feet. Have you ever seen a horse in the wild with metal shoes? I don't think so. There is nothing more important to a prey animal than good feet. And ours have helped us survive for millions and millions of years. Rock crushing hard and healthy.

But once upon a time, back in medieval days, some king decided he would be safer if he built his castle and fortress up on top of a high hill or mountain top. He still needed us to fight his wars, and move things and people around, but up there on top of the hill, there were no pastures like down in the valley. So he put us in small holding pens where we had to stand around all day, in our own pee and poop, and guess what happened to our feet. It wasn't the moisture so much as the ammonia. Ate our feet up! So when they'd take us out onto those hard stone roads... well, you can imagine.

The king's blacksmith came up with the idea of nailing metal shoes on to our hooves, to keep them from disintegrating when pounding the stony roads. There was a much simpler, healthier solution, but, unfortunately, it escaped the king and his blacksmith. Then, all the king's men and all the king's horses went down the hill... and all the king's peasants, living in the valley, where their horses were out in the field, happy as clams with strong and healthy hooves, saw these shiny, newfangled pieces of metal on the king's horses, and what did they say? Surely the king knows best! We must have some of those shiny metal things for our own horses!

And so it went for generations.

You humans are funny that way. And you say we follow the herd.

Joe and I have had long discussions about all this and he seems to be getting it. So I can shamelessly recommend his writings. Joe has spent much of his life trying to lure you into the heart and soul of a dog and now he's trying to lure you into the heart and soul of a horse. For it is there that he first began to comprehend the vast differences between us and you, and the kind of thinking that can bridge that gap and bind us together in relationship. My herd mates and I have taught him well. And, believe it or not, the philosophy behind everything he has learned doesn't just apply to horses, but to how you humans approach life as well. So whether or not you have a relationship with a horse, I think you'll find his journey of discovery fascinating.

I did.

And I already knew the story.

The comic strip character Pogo once said, "We have found the enemy and it is us." The problem with most issues concerning horses, we discovered, is not the horse, it's us. But I try to always remember that information is king. Following this chapter you will find links to all sorts of Resources and books that will provide you with more medical, technical, compassionate, and emotional material than you will ever need to prove to yourself that:

1. Horses have one of the best thermo-regulatory systems in the world. In virtually any climate and any geographical region their systems have more than what's needed to maintain their core body temperature at 38 degrees Celsius. "Blankets are a thermoregulatory nightmare for horses," says Dr. Hiltrud Strasser. Blankets prevent a horse from properly growing a winter coat, and when stripped of his blanket to ride in winter, he will not be prepared to protect himself against the low temperatures. Again, it's an issue fostered by humans. Winter is cold for us and we bundle up, so we think it must be logical that bundling up should be good for horses as well, when, in reality, it's the worst thing we can do. Same is true of heated and cooled barns and stables. Another issue (very logical actually) with blankets is that they only cover part of the body, and, within the horses system, in order to warm any part of the body, all the body must be warmed, thus some part is destined to be too hot or too cold, robbing the horse of its natural, complex, and highly efficient thermoregulatory system.

2., The blood vessels in the lower leg are very small in diameter when the horse is at rest, which is when leg wraps are put on, snugly, tightly. Then the horse begins to move, usually a lot, and the vessels need to increase their diameter to sufficiently circulate enough blood in the lower leg and hoof and return it to the heart, but this increased circulation is inhibited by the constricting wraps. There are also tendon issues. Dr. Strasser, in her book *A Lifetime of Soundness*, has several pages on this. Also, I have heard from many vets who have said the wraps do not give any real protection for the leg, except, perhaps, preventing a nick or two if one hoof hits another leg. So if you must use them, keep them loose so the vessels in the leg can expand and contract. Again, information is king.

3. Horses in the wild did just fine without metal shoes nailed on their feet for something like 50 million years before humans got hold of them. As a prey animal, a flight animal, they would've been extinct eons ago if they didn't know how to grow rock-solid feet that could run from predators and travel 8-20 miles a day in search of food and water. Still, more often than not, when I ask folks why they have shoes on their horses, the answers come back, "Well, it's always been done that way." When I press, it goes something like this:

"I guess it's because the hooves are not strong enough without them."

"Why," I ask.

"I don't know," they usually say.

"Don't you think you should know?" I ask.

"Well," they shrug, "everybody else has shoes. So it must be right."

And the reality is: it isn't.

Not even close to right.

4. Your horse should be turned out 24/7. No box stalls, however fancy and well equipped. You cannot imagine the stress this causes your horse, which in turn causes all sorts of medical and emotional problems.

So, Joe… are you saying that my horse needs thousands of acres to run around with other horses, and must travel ten to fifteen miles every day? Not at all. But replicating that lifestyle is not problematic as you might think. Our first two turnouts in California were each not much bigger than a barn. Steep and rocky. We mucked the turnouts twice a day and the hay is scattered, at ground level (which is how a horse was meant to eat, neck stretched to the ground) in at least twenty separate small piles around the turnout so the horses are in movement throughout the day, moving from one pile to another. With all that movement (and blood circulation increase) their previously shod feet became sound and strong so quickly it was astounding. We had two horses in one turnout and three in the other, so the five were constantly together. Then all of them moved to a similar pasture, approximately an acre, very steep and rocky, again, with their hay being scattered all around the pasture. Now in more than 100 little piles.

5. Ride bareback, at least some of the time.

Some of the most fun we and our horses have together is riding bareback usually with nothing more than a halter and looped lead rope. In less than a year, we have brought all of our horses up to be so responsive, trusting and caring about our desires, that truly they perform way better in a halter than they do in a bridle and bit. And they love bareback because they don't have the weight of the saddle and they can feel our bodies, and we can feel theirs. Whether you're trying to have more body/leg contact with your horse, or improve the balance point of your seat, or just have a quick ride without the hassle of tacking up, bareback is terrific, for both of you. And learn to train your horse so that your reins are always loose, preferably bitless, not tugging on your horses mouth. Teach your horse to do your bidding because it's his choice, not because you are forcing him by tugging on a bit. Google Stacy Westfall videos on YouTube and get inspired as she wins a reining competition with no bridle or saddle at all!

Not long ago, Kathleen would not even think of getting on a horse bareback, and now she rides more bareback than with a saddle. Feeling your horse and how she moves and she reacts to your various body positions and cues gives such a better understanding to what you need to do when in the saddle. Obviously, you should be careful, and go no faster than your seat is comfortable with, and if you haven't done the Beginning Groundwork to insure that you and your horse have a trusting partnership, that needs to be done first.

But when you're ready, riding bareback can truly enhance your overall horsemanship. Again, once you've
started, get a copy of Stacy Westfall's DVD and learn
how to do a complete reining demo with no bridle, no
halter, and no saddle. Amazing!

6. Train through relationship first.

We began our journey gobbling up the terrific material of renowned trainers and clinicians like Monty
Roberts, Charles Wilhelm, Clinton Anderson, John
Lyons, Stacy Westfall, Pat and Linda Parelli, Allen
Pogue, and natural hoof care specialists like Pete
Ramey, Eddie Drabek, and Jaime Jackson. Gobbling
up, in effect, hundreds of years of experience in a very
short time. And sorting through their methods, apply-
ing the best of what works for us. Every day I'm
amazed at how far one horse or the other has come and
all it takes is some knowledge, focus, and time. And
beginning with relationship first is a must. Then Leadership through ground work. Then working at liberty.
And suddenly your life with your horse has changed for
the better, better, better! It's really that simple. Stacy
Westfall recently said that the best thing she has ever
done for her training is to do no training until the relationship is right.

During our first year on this journey, I trailered one
of our horses across town, a horse who came to us five
months before, green broke with very little mileage and
not much ground work. But he learned to focus with a

capital F. He caught his foot in the hay feeder in the trailer and, as I entered the trailer to unload him, he freaked out completely. Imagine being in a trailer with a horse used to four legs having only three. But instead of winding up in the hospital, I wound up with his leg out of the hay feeder, with him focused on me, paying strict attention, even though his eyes were glazed and his nostrils flared. He listened, he backed, he yielded, and allowed me to walk calmly out of the trailer first, with him following... calmly. The entire story is told in *The Soul of a Horse*. But it's all about ground work. This, with Join Up, is the foundation we worked on with each of our horses.

We started on the ground, getting to know our horses and what makes them tick, and establishing a real relationship. Giving them the choice of whether they want to be with us or not. A horse is not a motorcycle but is a living, breathing, fearful flight animal who needs and wants a good leader and friend. We believe in beginning a horse so that he will learn without fear, be safe, be attentive and desirous to please, and will be well prepared for a long and happy relationship. His choice. That's the important part. That's what changes everything. Our horses range in age from baby to twenty-five, but they all began with us (or are beginning with us) the same way, and have been brought along the same way. It's truly amazing to watch an older, well-schooled horse re-learn everything and become a willing and desirous partner and friend.

Not long ago we were scared out of our minds by these 1000-pound animals. We aren't multiple-time world champions or thirty year veterans, but Kathleen and I have had the benefit of more amazing experts than you've ever found in one place before. Our goal is to inspire you to learn, and apply, and trust yourself enough to let your horses be your teachers, to figure things out instead of clinging to "somebody else's "paint by numbers" horsemanship. And to discover the pure joy of seeing that something so simple actually works.

Discovering the mysteries of the horse is a never-ending journey, but the rewards are an elixir. The soul prospers from sharing, caring, relating, and fulfilling. Nothing can make you feel better than doing something good for another being. Not cars. Not houses. Not facelifts. Not blue ribbons or trophies. And there is nothing more important in life than love. Not money. Not status. Not winning.

Try it and you will understand what I mean. Apply it to your horses, and your life. It is the synthesis of our books and why they came into being.

Give the choice of *choice*. Care enough to want your horses to be healthy and happy. Care enough to remove the stress from their lives. It will come back a hundredfold.

And always question everything. Be your own expert. Gather information and make decisions based upon knowledge and wisdom, not hearsay or convenience. Know that if something doesn't seem logical, it probably isn't. If it doesn't make sense, it's probably not right.

Learn the art of discipline with compassion.

And care about the way we care for the domestic horse. It needs to change. An extreme makeover, if you will. Going back to square one and beginning anew to remove the unnecessary stress from their lives. Because removing that stress also removes illnesses, hoof problems, and behavior problems. And creates a happy horse who wants to be a willing partner.

I'm still astonished when I think where Kathleen and I began such a short time ago, and where most horse owners still are today, training with dominance if not cruelty, cooping up their horses in small spaces, weakening their natural immune systems, feeding them unnaturally, creating unhealthy hooves and bodies with metal shoes. All because most folks actually believe it's the right thing to do.

Yes, there are some who still only want a beast of burden. *Do as I say. Make me a winner. Jump higher. Run faster. Slide farther.* People who care not about having a relationship with their horse, and who will, when confronted, continue to care not about the health and happiness of their horse. But I believe that most horse owners today care about their horses and are operating, as we once were, with little more than emotional logic, old wives' tales, and very little real knowledge. I hope this book will be a crack in the armor, a small breeze if not the strong winds of change, a resource for what needs to be done.

And a longer, happier, healthier life for all horses.

Follow Joe & Kathleen's Journey
From no horses and no clue to stumbling through
mistakes, fear, fascination and frustration on a collision
course with the ultimate discovery that something was
very wrong in the world of horses.

Read the National Best Seller
The Soul of a Horse
Life Lessons from the Herd

...and the Highly Acclaimed Best Selling Sequel

Born Wild
The Soul of a Horse

*The above links and all of the links that follow are live links in
the eBook editions available at Amazon Kindle, Barnes & Noble
Nook, and Apple iBooks*

Also by Joe Camp

What Readers and Critics Are Saying About Joe Camp

"Joe Camp is a master storyteller." - *THE NEW YORK TIMES*

"Joe Camp is a natural when it comes to understanding how animals tick and a genius at telling us their story. His books are must-reads for those who love animals of any species." - *MONTY ROBERTS, AUTHOR OF NEW YORK TIMES BEST-SELLER THE MAN WHO LISTENS TO HORSES*

"The tightly written, simply designed, and powerfully drawn chapters often read like short stories that flow from the heart. Camp has become something of a master at telling us what can be learned from animals, in this case specifically horses, without making us realize we have been educated, and, that is, perhaps, the mark of a real teacher." - *JACK L. KENNEDY, THE JOPLIN INDEPENDENT*

"One cannot help but be touched by Camp's love and sympathy for animals and by his eloquence on the subject." - *MICHAEL KORDA, THE WASHINGTON POST*

"Joe Camp is a gifted storyteller and the results are magical. Joe entertains, educates and empowers, baring his own soul while articulating keystone principles of a modern revolution in horsemanship." - *RICK LAMB, AUTHOR AND TV/RADIO HOST "THE HORSE SHOW"*

FIVE UNDENIABLE TRUTHS

One: The first Undeniable Truth – Science tells us that it would take a minimum of 5000 years – probably closer to 10,000 – to even begin to change the base genetics of any species. In other words, no matter what anyone tells you to the contrary, a few hundred years of selective breeding has no effect on base genetics whatsoever or the horse's ability to grow the kind of rock solid foot he was born to have. This is the foundation for all that follows. Everything begins right here. The wild horse in the western high desert of the United States has incredible feet. He must have to escape predators and to search for food and water. If he didn't have incredible feet he'd be extinct. We would have never known him. And the wild horse and the domestic horse of today are genetically exactly the same. The domestic horse's foot is not genetically weak and unhealthy. Not even the oft-claimed Thoroughbred. The conditions under which any horse lives can certainly cause ill health, but the horse's genetics can fix that, given the opportunity.

Two: DNA sequencing was done on bones of horses discovered in the Alaskan permafrost dating 12,000 to 28,000 years old... and this DNA sequencing was compared to DNA sequencing from today's domestic horse... and there was less than 1.2% difference in those 28,000 year old horses and the horse in your back yard. Documented and on record. Confirming, once again, that the base genetics of every horse on the planet are the same. Science confirms for us that every horse on this earth "retains the ability to return successfully to the wild or feral state" – note that they say *successfully* – and that includes growing himself or herself a great foot that would protect this flight animal from predators and give him – or her – the ability to travel 8-20 miles every day of his life.

Three: The horse began and evolved for 50+ million years in and around the Great Basin of the western United States... then he crossed the Bering Straits Land Bridge into Siberia spreading into the rest of the world. Which means that the horse – as we know it today – spent 50+ million years evolving – now please get this because it's important – the horse spent 50+ million years evolving to live in conditions and on terrain like the western high desert of the United States and no horse will ever adapt to the terrain and environment in our new home in middle Tennessee...or at least not for 5000 to 10,000 years... and it is therefore up to us – Kathleen and myself – to do everything within our power to replicate the lifestyle they would be living if they were living in the great basin – which is effectively the lifestyle they were living at our high desert home in southern California before moving to middle Tennessee.

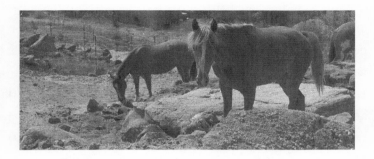

The herd in California

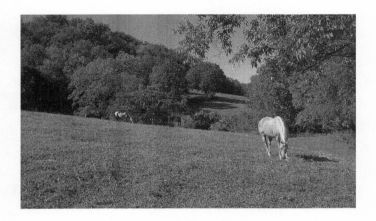

The herd in Tennessee

Four: Undeniable Truth #4 (or perhaps #1): a horse's hoof is supposed to flex with every impact of the ground. Every time it hits the ground it flexes outward – like a toilet plunger – and then snaps back when the hoof comes off the ground. That flexing sucks an enormous amount of blood into the hoof mechanism...

keeps it healthy, helps it to grow properly, helps fight off problems... AND all that liquid provides an hydraulic-like shock absorption for the joints, ligaments, and tendons of the leg. Wow... who knew? At one point I remember believing the horse's hoof was just a wad of hard stuff... like one big fingernail.

But there's more. When the foot lifts off the ground and the flexed hoof snaps back, the power of that contraction shoves the blood in the hoof capsule back up those long skinny legs, taking strain off the heart.

So what happens to all this good stuff when a metal shoe is nailed to the hoof?

Nothing.

No circulation (or substantially reduced circulation)... no shock absorption (in fact if you've ever seen the videos of the vibrations set off up the leg when a metal shoe slams into the ground see link below, it'll freak you out)... and no assistance to the heart in getting that blood back up the leg.

Five: There is no hoof lameness in the wild (the wild of the American west where the horse evolved for 50+ million years; the terrain he is well used to living on). Yet the American Farriers Association reports that 95% of domestic horses have some degree of hoof lameness? Some folks want to say that's because the domestic hoof is inherently weak. But as we've already established, the inherent genetics are the same as the wild horse. The reasons for so much domestic hoof lameness are the metal shoes, diet, lifestyle, stress, and in some cases work load that we have forced upon the horse. In other words: No Stalls, no shoes, no sugar! In simple terms, what all this means is that a horse's entire physiology has been built over millions of years to:

One: Move a minimum of 8 to 20 miles a day, <u>on bare hooves</u>.

Two: Be with a herd, and thus physically and emotionally safe, unstressed.

Three: Spend 16 to 18 hours a day eating… <u>from the ground</u>, a variety, but mostly grass or grass hay; a continuous uptake in small quantities to suit their small tummies and the function of their hindguts.

Four: Control their own thermoregulatory system, thus controlling their own internal body temperature with no outside assistance, including heat, blankets, and the like.

Five: Stand and walk on firm fresh ground, not in the chemical remnants of their own poop and pee… nor be breathing the fumes of those remnants, plus the excessive carbon dioxide that accumulates inside a closed structure. In other words, no stalls.

Six: Get a certain amount of unstressed REM sleep, which requires them to lie down, which will usually only happen when our in the company of other horses, for guard duty.

RESOURCES

There are, I'm certain, many programs and people who subscribe to these philosophies and are very good at what they do but are not listed in these resources. That's because we haven't experienced them, and we will only recommend to you programs that we believe, from our own personal experience, to be good for the horse and well worth the time and/or money. First I've listed a few links from our website and blog that relate to what you've just read:

Our No Agenda Time
http://thesoulofahorse.com/blog/no-agenda-time-join-up-without-a-round-pen/

Happier Healthier Horses Around the World
http://thesoulofahorse.com/blog/powerful-stories-from-happier-healthier-horses/

Photos of Barefoot Champions
http://thesoulofahorse.com/blog/barefoot-champions/

Diet: A Slippery Slope
http://thesoulofahorse.com/a-slippery-slope/

Video of Joe and Cash: Relationship First!
Go to: http://www.youtube.com/user/thesoulofahorse
Then scroll down to Relationship First

Video: Finding The Soul of a Horse
http://www.youtube.com/user/thesoulofahorse

Video: Don't Ask for Patience – God
Will Give You a Horse
Go to: http://www.youtube.com/user/thesoulofahorse
Then scroll down to Relationship First

<u>**Taking Your Horse Barefoot:**</u> Taking your horses barefoot involves more than just pulling shoes. The new breed of natural hoof care practitioners have studied and rely completely on what they call the **wild horse model,** which replicates the trim that horses give to themselves in the wild through natural wear. The more the domesticated horse is out and about, moving constantly, the less trimming he or she will need. The more stall-bound the horse, the more trimming will be needed in order to keep the hooves healthy and in shape. Every horse is a candidate to live as nature intended. The object is to maintain their hooves as if they were in the wild, and that requires some study. Not a lot, but definitely some. I now consider myself capable of keeping my horses' hooves in shape over a short period of time. I don't do their regular trim, but I do perform in-

terim touch-ups. I prefer to have someone who sees hundreds of horses' hooves every week. The myth that domesticated horses *must* wear shoes has been proven to be pure hogwash. The fact that shoes degenerate the health of the hoof and the entire horse has not only been proven, but is also recognized even by those who nail shoes on horses. Successful high performance bare-footedness with the wild horse trim can be accomplished for virtually every horse on the planet, and the process has even been proven to be a healing procedure for horses with laminitis, founder, navicular, ertc. On this subject, I beg you not to wait. Dive into the material below and give your horse a longer, healthier, happier life.

http://www.hoofrehab.com/– This is Pete Ramey's website. If you read only one book on this entire subject, read Pete's *Making Natural Hoof Care Work for You.* Or better yet, get his DVD series *Under the Horse,* which is fourteen-plus hours of terrific research, trimming, and information. If you've ever doubted the fact that horses do not need metal shoes and are in fact better off without them, please go to Pete's website. He will convince you otherwise. Then use his teachings to guide your horses' venture into barefootedness. He is never afraid or embarrassed to change his opinion on something as he learns more from his experiences. Pete's writings have also appeared in *Horse & Rider* and are on his website. He has taken all of Clinton Anderson's horses barefoot.

http://www.paddockparadise.com/ - This is Jaime Jackson's website. Jaime is more or less the father of natural hoof care in the United States. He has studied and photographed the hooves of more than a thousand wild horses, hooves that are amazingly similar, no matter the variances in geography and climate. Rock solid, concave, beveled on the edges, and as healthy as can be. His book *Horse Owners Guide to Natural Hoof Care* is the "bible" and should be read. If you truly want to learn all you can learn about this subject, read both Jaime's book and Pete's, beginning with Jaime's. Pete even lists Jaime's book as a prerequisite to his. That said, this book also goes deeply into Jaime's research of the wild horse hoof and why this trim can work for any horse. For me, this was all fascinating material.

The following are other websites that contain good information regarding the barefoot subject:

http://www.wholehorsetrim.com - This is the website of Eddie Drabek, another one of my heroes. Eddie is a wonderful trimmer in Houston, Texas, and an articulate and inspirational educator and spokesman for getting metal shoes off horses. Read everything he has written, including the pieces on all the horses whose lives he has saved by taking them barefoot.

http://www.TheHorsesHoof.com – this website and magazine of Yvonne and James Welz is devoted entirely to barefoot horses around the world and is surely the single largest resource for owners, trimmers, case histories, and virtually everything you would ever want to know about barefoot horses. With years and years of barefoot experience, Yvonne is an amazing resource. She can compare intelligently this method vs that and help you to understand all there is to know. And James is a super barefoot trimmer.

Our current hoof specialist in Tennessee is Mark Taylor who works in Tennessee, Arkansas, Alabama, and Mississippi 662-224-4158
http://www.barefoothorsetrimming.com/

http://www.aanhcp.net_- This is the website for the American Association of Natural Hoof Care Practioners.

Also see at
http://www.youtube.com/user/thesoulofahorse
Then scroll down to the video title

Video of Joe: Why Are Our Horses Barefoot?

Video: The Soul of a Horse Paddock Paradise: What We Did, How We Did It, and Why

Video of Joe: Why Our Horses Eat from the Ground

The next 2 titles at the are very short slow-motion videos of a horse's hoof hitting the ground. One is a shod hoof, one is barefoot. Watch the vibrations roll up the leg from the shod hoof... then imagine that happening every time any shod hoof hits the ground. Go to:

http://www.youtube.com/user/thesoulofahorse
Then scroll way down to the video titles

Video: Trotting Shod Hoof
Video: Trotting Barefoot Hoof

Find a recommended trimmer in your area:

http://www.liberatedhorsemanship.com/Liberated_Horsemanship_Home.html

http://www.aanhcp.net/

http://www.americanhoofassociation.org/

http://www.pacifichoofcare.org/

Here's a link to a terrific article on the Houston Mounted Patrol's total conversion to barefoot; all forty or so of their horses now work downtown Houston's concrete, asphalt, and marble completely barefoot: http://thesoulofahorse.com/city-of-houston-police-horses-all-barefoot/

Natural Boarding: Once your horses are barefoot, please begin to figure out how to keep them out around the clock, day and night, moving constantly, or at least having that option. It's really not as difficult as you might imagine, even if you only have access to a small piece of property. Every step your horse takes makes his hooves and his body healthier, his immune system better. And it really is not that difficult or expensive to figure it out. Much cheaper than barns and stalls.

Paddock Paradise: A Guide to Natural Horse Boarding This book by Jaime Jackson begins with a study of horses in the wild, then describes many plans for getting your horses out 24/7, even if your property is very small, in replication of the wild. The designs are all very specific, but by reading the entire book you begin to deduce what's really important and what's not so important, and why. We didn't follow any of his plans, but we have one pasture that's probably an acre and a half and two much smaller ones (photos on our website and see the video below). All of them function very well when combined with random food placement. They keep our horses on the move, as they would be in the wild. The big one is very inexpensively electrically-fenced. *Paddock Paradise* is available, as are all of Jaime's books, at **http://www.paddockparadise.com/**

Also at **http://www.youtube.com/user/thesoulofahorse**
And scroll down to:
Video: The Soul of a Horse Paddock Paradise: What We Did, How We Did It, and Why
and
Video of Joe: Why Our Horses Eat from the Ground

New resources are regularly updated on Kathleen's and Joe's: **www.theSoulofaHorse.com** or their blog **http://thesoulofahorse.com/blog**

Valuable Links on Diet and Nutrition:

Dr. Juliette Getty's website:
http://gettyequinenutrition.biz/

Dr. Getty's favorite feed/forage testing facility:
Equi-Analytical Labs:
http://www.equi-analytical.com

The Diet page on our website:
http://thesoulofahorse.com/a-slippery-slope/

<u>Natural Horsemanship</u>: Natural Horsemanship is the current buzz word for those who train horses or teach humans the training of horses without any use of fear,

cruelty, threats, aggression, or pain. The philosophy is growing like wildfire, and why shouldn't it? If you can accomplish everything you could ever hope for with your horse and still have a terrific relationship with him or her, and be respected as a leader, not feared as a dominant predator, why wouldn't you? As with any broadly based general philosophy, there are many differing schools of thought on what is important and what isn't, what works well and what doesn't. Which of these works best for you, I believe, depends a great deal on how you learn, and how much reinforcement and structure you need. Our beginning is more or less a shuffling together of the first three below whose websites are listed, favoring one source for this and another for that. Often, this gives us an opportunity to see how different programs handle the same topic, which enriches insight. But, ultimately, they all end up at the same place: When you have a good relationship with your horse that began with the horse's choice, when you are respected as your horse's leader, when you truly care for your horse, then, before too long, you will be able to figure out for yourself the best communication to evoke any particular objective. These programs, as written, or taped on DVD, merely give you a structured format to follow that will take you to that goal.

Monty Roberts and Join up:

http://www.montyroberts.com- Start here, please. Or at Monty's Equus Online University which is terrific and probably the best Equine learning value out there on the internet. Learn Monty's Join-Up method. Watching his *Join-Up* DVD was probably our single most pivotal experience. Even if you've owned your horse forever, go back to the beginning and watch this DVD (or watch it Join-Up at his Online University), then do it yourself with your horse or horses. You'll find that when you unconditionally offer choice to your horse and he chooses you, everything changes. You become a member of the herd, and your horse's leader, and with that goes responsibility on his part as well as yours. Even if you don't own horses, it is absolutely fascinating to watch Monty put a saddle and a rider on a completely unbroken horse in less than thirty minutes (unedited!). In the beginning we also watched and used Monty's *Dually Training Halter* DVD and his *Load-Up trailering* DVD. And we loved his books: *The Man Who Listens to Horses, The Horses in My Life, From My Hands to Yours, and Shy Boy*. Monty is a very impressive man who cares a great deal for horses.

http://www.parelli.com_- Pat and Linda Parelli have turned their teaching methods into a fully accredited college curriculum. We have four of their home DVD courses: *Level 1, Level 2, Level 3*, and *Liberty & Horse Behavior*. We recommend them all, but especially the first three. Often, they do run on, dragging out points much longer than perhaps necessary, but we've found, particularly in the early days, that knowledge gained through such saturation always bubbles up to present itself at the most opportune moments. In other words, it's good. Soak it up. It'll pay dividends later. Linda is a good instructor, especially in the first three programs, and Pat is one of the most amazing horsemen I've ever seen. His antics are inspirational for me. Not that I will ever duplicate many of them, but knowing that it's possible is very affirming. Pat's 17-minute demonstration teaching Games 2, 3, and 4 to a new untrained horse on DVD #2 of their Level 1 Kit was worth the price of the entire set. Virtually everything you need to know about groundwork in 17 minutes. Soak this man up anytime you can. And watching him with a newborn foal is just fantastic. The difficulty for us with *Liberty & Horse Behavior* (besides its price) is on disk 5 whereon Linda consumes almost three hours to load an inconsistent horse into a trailer. Her belief is that the horse should *not* be *made* to do anything, he should *discover* it on his own. I believe there's another option. As Monty Roberts teaches, there is a big difference between *making* a horse do something and *leading* him through it, showing him that it's okay, that his trust in you is valid. Once you have joined up with him, and he trusts you, he is willing to take chances for you because of that trust, so long as you don't abuse the trust. On Monty's trailer-loading DVD Monty takes about one-tenth the time, and the horse (who was impossible to load before Monty) winds up loading himself from thirty feet away, happily, even playfully. And his trust in Monty has progressed as well, because he reached beyond his comfort zone and learned it was okay. His trust was confirmed. And I've never seen Pat Parelli take longer than maybe 30 minutes to teach a horse to load. One thing the Parelli program stresses, in a way, is a follow up to Monty Roberts' Join-Up: you should spend a lot of time just hanging out with your horse. In the stall, in the pasture, wherever. Quality time, so to speak. No agenda, just hanging out. Very much a relationship enhancer. And don't ever stomp straight over to your horse and slap on a halter. Wait. Let your horse come to you. It's that choice thing again, and Monty or Pat and Linda Parelli can teach you how it works.

http://www.downunderhorsemanship.com -
This is Clinton Anderson's site. Whereas the Parellis are very philosophically oriented, Clinton gets down to business with lots of detail and repetition. What exactly do I do to get my horse to back up? From the ground and from the saddle, he shows you precisely, over and over again. And when you're in the arena or round pen and forget whether he used his left hand or right hand, or whether his finger was pointing up or down, it's very easy to go straightaway to the answer on his DVDs. His

programs are very task-oriented, and, again, there are a bunch of them. We have consumed his *Gaining Respect and Control on the Ground, Series I through III* and *Riding with Confidence, Series I through III*. And his new *Fundamentals* program. All are multiple DVD sets, so there has been a lot of viewing and reviewing. For the most part, his tasks and the Parellis are much the same, though usually the teaching is approached very differently. Both have served a purpose for us. We also loved his *No Worries Tying DVD* for use with his Australian Tie Ring, which truly eliminates pull-back problems in minutes! And on this one he demonstrates terrific desensitizing techniques. Clinton is a two-time winner of the Road to the Horse competition, in which three top natural-horsemanship clinicians are given unbroken horses and a mere three hours to be riding and performing specified tasks. Those DVDs are terrific! And Clinton's Australian accent is also fun to listen to... mate.

The three programs above have built our natural horsemanship foundation, and we are in their debt. The following are a few others you should probably check out, each featuring a highly respected clinician, and all well known for their care and concern for horses.

http://www.imagineahorse.com_- This is Allen Pogue and Suzanne De Laurentis' site. Allen's work has unfortunately cast him as a trick trainer, but it's so much more than that. We've just recently discovered Allen and are dumbfounded by how his horses treat him and try for him. His work with young horses is so logical and powerful that you should study it even if you never intend to own a horse. Allen says "With my young horses, by the time they are three years old they are so mentally mature that saddling and a short ride is absolutely undramatic." He has taken Dr. Robert M. Miller's book *Imprint Training of the Newborn Foal* to a new and exponential level.

http://www.robertmmiller.com - Dr. Robert M. Miller is an equine veterinarian and world renowned speaker and author on horse behavior and natural horsemanship. I think his name comes up more often in these circles than anyone else's. His first book, *Imprint Training of the Newborn Foal* is now a bible of the horse world. He's not really a trainer, per se, but a phenomenal resource on horse behavior. He will show you the route to "the bond." You must visit his website.

http://www.chrislombard.com/ - An amazing horseman and wonderful teacher. His DVD *Beginning with the Horse* puts relationship, leadership and trust into simple easy-to-understand terms. And only one DVD :).

Frederick Pignon – This man is amazing and has taken relationship and bond with his horses to an astounding new level. Go to this link:
http://www.youtube.com/watch?v=w1YO3j-Zh3g
and watch the video of his show with three beautiful black Lusitano stallions, all at liberty. This show would border on the miraculous if they were all geldings, but they're not. They're stallions. Most of us will never achieve the level of bond Frederick has achieved with his horses but it's inspiring to know that it's possible, and to see what the horse-human relationship is capable of becoming. Frederick believes in true partnership with his horses, he believes in making every training session fun not work, he encourages the horses to offer their ideas, and he uses treats. And when he begins a performance he says that he never knows exactly where it's going to go. When Kathleen read his book *Gallop to Freedom* her response to me was simply, "Can we just move in with them?"

For more about pretty much anything in this book please visit one of these websites:

thesoulofahorse.com

www.14handspress.com

The Soul of a Horse Fan Page on Facebook
https://www.facebook.com/pages/The-Soul-of-a-Horse/106606472709815

The Soul of a Horse Channel on YouTube
http://www.youtube.com/user/thesoulofahorse

Joe and The Soul of a Horse on Twitter
https://twitter.com/Joe_camp

Again, all of the links above and throughout this book are live links on the eBook editions available at Amazon Kindle, Barnes & Noble Nook, and Apple iBooks

16163170R00081

Made in the USA
San Bernardino, CA
21 October 2014